From Midnight

To Daylight

An Inspiring Autobiography

by

Brenda E. Rocker

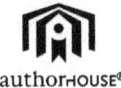
authorHOUSE®

AuthorHouse™
1663 Liberty Drive, Suite 200
Bloomington, IN 47403
www.authorhouse.com
Phone: 1-800-839-8640

First published by AuthorHouse 9/24/2010

ISBN: 978-1-4389-1268-4 (sc)
ISBN: 978-1-4389-1267-7 (hc)

Printed in the United States of America
Bloomington, Indiana

This book is printed on acid-free paper.

From Midnight to Daylight

is dedicated in memory of my sisters around the world that lost their battle to breast cancer. I promise that your death will not be in vain, and that I will work diligently in spreading the word "Early detection is the key to life." Rest in peace my sisters, and your memories will always have a special place in my heart.

Without God in my life, I would not exist. I called upon Him, and He answered my prayers.

Table of Contents

Acknowledgements

To MY BEST FRIEND, KIM Taylor, who is now with our Lord, I love you, and my happiness is owed to you.

To my parents, Don L. and Ella Mae Anderson, your love and support will remain close to my heart. To my siblings, Ethel, Cornelius, Beverly, Natalie, Ronald, and Kimberly, thanks for supporting me in my decision to write this book.

To my cousin Derrick (Tyrone) Simpson, thanks for the many years of love and support. Your love will always hold a special place in my heart.

I give thanks to God for sending me three "guardian angels" to watch over me. Dr. James Lawrence, Dr. William Thomas, and Dr. Gaylord Walker, your wisdom has given me the hope and the courage to survive. I will forever remember my "guardian angels" sent from heaven.

Introduction

My FIRST EXPERIENCE WITH BREAST cancer was in 1987. I discovered a painful lump located in my left breast while undressing. I was terrified of the possibility of breast cancer because of the history of the disease in my family. I immediately called my mother, who suggested I make an appointment for a mammogram. I took her advice and called the medical center the following morning to schedule an appointment.

I left the house early the day of my appointment, being a first-time patient, I would have plenty of documents to complete. I felt dazed, as if I were in a trance, and everything appeared to be in slow motion. As I waited to be called, my heart was racing, and I could feel the anxiety building up and taking control. Every dreadful scenario I could imagine entered my mind. I sat there in disbelief, wondering how this could be happening. I was only twenty-eight years old—too young to have breast cancer.

Finally, my name was called and I was led down the hallway to an examining room. The nurse asked several mandatory questions pertaining to my health and my family's medical history. Once she finished her questions, I was given a gown and asked to remove my top; she informed me the doctor would be in shortly.

It felt as if an eternity had passed before the doctor and nurse entered the room. He introduced himself and asked what problems was I experiencing. I explained that while recently getting undressed, I had discovered a lump in my left breast that was extremely painful at the time. He asked me to lie down so he could examine me to better assess the situation. Upon his examination, he discovered my breasts were large. He then educated me regarding a condition called lumpy breast. Lumpy breast condition occurs when the breast tissue develops in lumps, but are not cancerous.

When the doctor concluded his examination, he suggested I have a specialist on staff examine me to be positive of the lumpy breast condition. I agreed, so he notified the specialist. The specialist entered the room ten minutes later and introduced himself. He asked if he could examine me. After his examination, he also concluded that my breasts were large and that more than likely, I did indeed have the lumpy breast condition.

Both doctors recommended I have a mammogram to ensure the lumps were not cancer related. I was taken to radiology for my first mammogram, which was painful, but it only lasted a few minutes. After the x-rays, I returned to the examining room and waited patiently for the results.

Finally, both doctors entered the room and confirmed there were no signs of breast cancer. However, they suggested it would be an excellent idea for me to start having yearly mammograms, because in some cases, women diagnosed with lumpy breast had developed breast cancer in their later years.

I was elated regarding the mammogram results. When I arrived home, I immediately called my mother and informed her of the astonishing news. My life appeared to be normal again; the clouds had been lifted, and I was looking forward to a beautiful day.

Chapter One:

Dealing With Breast Cancer

IT HAD BEEN A YEAR since my mammogram examination, and my twenty-ninth birthday was approaching. I decided it was time to schedule an appointment for an annual mammogram and pap smear. To my surprise, every clinic I contacted said I was too young to have a mammogram and suggested I wait until at least my thirty-fifth birthday.

Finally, the last clinic I called agreed once I explained the lumpy breast incident and my family history of breast cancer. The appointment was scheduled several days before my birthday.

My persistence had paid off. For the next nine years, I scheduled my annual mammograms and pap smears around my birthday, and the results were always negative. However, in 1991, I became ill and was diagnosed with lupus. Lupus is an autoimmune disease (blood disease) that causes rheumatoid arthritis, fatigue, sickness, and a butterfly rash that appears across the bridge of the nose and both cheeks. At the present time there are no cures, but there are medications that can control the disease. I have learned to manage my lupus by living a stress-free life to the best of my ability.

I thank God that my good days outnumber the bad ones.

In 1996, I was blessed with the opportunity of owning a restaurant, which has always been a dream of mine. I was contemplating operating a deli that caters to the lunch crowd located in a small business district. There were at least one thousand potential customers, so I felt I should do well financially. Although a little apprehensive, I was up to the tremendous challenge that lay ahead of me.

After signing the lease I named the deli Mike's Deli, after my husband Michael. I was overjoyed at seeing my longtime vision becoming a reality. One of the most difficult challenges would be converting an office into a full-service restaurant. I placed the furniture order for the dinning room and office. The stove, refrigerator, and prep table were to be delivered later in the week on Thursday.

When the dinning room furniture arrived, I decorated the room to give it a masculine ambiance, as 75% of the employees in the area are men. The walls featured pictures of antique Ford cars and Arabian horses. Two six-foot fig trees adorned each side of the window, and tables were placed throughout the dining room. One could hear the sounds of jazz playing as it filled the air.

The food inventory was ordered early to guarantee everything would go smoothly for the grand opening, which was planned on Michael's birthday in June. My staff and I performed a trial run several days before the celebration to guarantee we could accommodate the influx of guests and customers participating in the celebration. We planned to serve every item on the menu, giving the guests and customers the opportunity to experience the varieties of delicacies available.

The grand opening was awesome. We had a magnificent turnout.

There were so many people present that we had to extend the hours of celebration to accommodate everyone. We received excellent reviews for the food presentation and atmosphere. My staff and I were exhausted, but I could not have asked for a more successful celebration.

After two months, we had established a lunch clientele, including a few regulars that patronized us daily. I must admit the deli was more difficult to manage than I had anticipated, but it was worth the time and energy invested each day.

One September evening, while lying in bed, I discovered a lump between my breast and ribcage. My instinct immediately told me it was breast cancer, and I instantly sentenced myself to death. Although the thoughts of having breast cancer terrified me, I did nothing to learn if the lump was breast cancer, perhaps thinking the lump would disappear.

However, in November I decided to share my discovery with Michael. He was horrified and wanted to know my plans. The possibility of me having breast cancer petrified him, and I still had not scheduled a mammogram.

My youngest sister, Kimberly, was graduating from Chicago State University with honors, and I wanted to be there to support her on her joyous and memorable occasion.

Kimberly's graduation was scheduled January 18, 1997, and I did not want to receive any disappointing news before we celebrated her accomplishments. However, I did schedule my mammogram for the end of January—two months earlier than my annual appointment in March.

Michael and I traveled to Chicago the Friday before graduation. The weather was atrocious, and it became worse as we approached Chicago Heights. Semi trucks and trailers were jackknifed all over the highway. At times, we could only travel 15 to 20 mph. At one time we considered turning back, but we decided to continue. When we finally arrived in Chicago Heights, it was twenty-two hours later; we were exhausted and just wanted to relax from the tiresome trip.

Saturday morning we were all excited for Kimberly. She had, without any doubts, earned her degree. Kimberly attended school on Tuesday and Thursday from 7:00 a.m. to 9:00 p.m. because of her family obligations—marriage and caring for two children. She was determined to achieve her educational goals. She was graduating with honors, magna cum laude, and she had earned a lifetime membership on the board of psychology and science. During the graduation ceremony, I cried tears of joy just knowing Kimberly could begin her new life. I decided to inform my family of my suspicion of breast cancer, after Kimberly's graduation. I knew I had to tell them soon, because in the morning we would be returning to Mobile.

After finally sharing my suspicions of breast cancer, everyone was shocked and filled with disbelief. They wanted to know when I had received the diagnosis. I informed them I had not seen my physician but was scheduled for an appointment January 29, 1997. They immediately thought I had lost my mind. Deep in my heart, I knew it was breast cancer.

I informed my mother of the possibility of having to come to Mobile, and I needed her to bring me a set of flannel pajamas when she came for my surgery. In Alabama, it's difficult to purchase flannel pajamas due to the mild winter months. She laughed and agreed. I knew she was just humoring me, and that's why she agreed to purchase two sets. After my announcement, Michael and I said goodnight; we turned in early to get an early start in the morning.

We left Chicago Heights Sunday morning. We stopped and had breakfast; then we headed down Interstate 65 South. Neither one of us was looking forward to the long, exhausting drive so soon, but it could not be avoided. We knew there would be beautiful weather with sunny skies once we made it to Tennessee . And we were anticipating the warmer weather. It is amazing how the climate changes dramatically when one travels only eight to ten hours south. When I lived in Chicago, I never gave winter a second thought; I simply acclimated and carried on.

The day of my clinic appointment had arrived. On my way to the clinic, I experienced déjà vu. Memories of the lumpy breast ordeal of 1987 flashed before my eyes. After entering the clinic, I signed into radiology and waited for my name to be called. The x-ray technician called me immediately. She handed me a gown and instructed me to get undressed from the waist up and have a seat behind the screen. She mentioned she would be with me soon.

At least fifteen minutes passed before my name was called. The x-ray technician explained the procedure. She then took several x–rays to guarantee she captured all dimensions of my breast. There was only a small amount of discomfort associated with the mammogram.

Once the mammogram was completed, I took a seat in the waiting area until the radiologist could read the x-rays. This appeared to be the longest wait of my life. Every dreadful scenario imaginable ran across my mind as I waited to be called.

I wanted to cry but fought back the tears, trying not to stress unnecessarily. The anxiety was building up in my chest. I prayed everything would be fine, although deep within my heart I knew the diagnosis would be breast cancer. I prayed for the strength to be courageous. At that moment I wished very badly Michael had accompanied me, but it was all too late. I was praying this nightmare would end soon.

It took half an hour for the x-rays to be read, and then the door to radiology opened, and there stood a tall male doctor in the doorway.

From the expression upon his face, I knew the mammogram was positive for breast cancer. He called my name and escorted me to his office. Once inside his office, he spoke those dreaded words I had feared hearing for months; I had breast cancer and needed to check myself into the hospital immediately. I panicked and screamed at him to get away from me. I was devastated.

My only instinct was to literally run out of the clinic, get into my car, and drive away. Before I realized it, I had driven home in only ten minutes, still in shock and wondering how this could be happening. I had never missed a mammogram checkup in ten years. Despair filled my mind. I could only wonder when the cancer had developed. I felt defenseless and hopeless; there wasn't anything I could do despite all my efforts to avoid this situation. I couldn't help but wonder why the cancer hadn't been detected on my mammogram from the previous year.

Shortly after arriving home, I received a telephone call from Memorial Medical Center. A soft-spoken nurse was on the other end. She said the cancer center had contacted them regarding my diagnosis. She emphasized the importance of my coming to the clinic for a biopsy. I agreed and asked when an appointment would be available, and she told me I could come in that day. I inquired about a time and asked for directions.

I arrived at the clinic still in shock and filled with disbelief. Upon entering the clinic, I immediately noticed the waiting area was empty. The nurse and the doctor were waiting for me. I filled out the necessary forms giving them consent to perform the biopsy. A few minutes passed before the nurse called my name.

She instructed me to get undressed and handed me a gown. I did as instructed, still in shock and completely numb.

I must admit my ignorance to what a biopsy involved. Dr. Osmont entered the room. He was in his early sixties, wore glasses, and had beautiful silver hair. He introduced himself and said he needed to perform a needle biopsy. I did not understand what the biopsy entailed until seeing the needle. The nurse realized the situation was unbearable; she held my hand and assured me everything would be over in a matter of minutes.

When Dr. Osmont inserted the needle into my breast, I became lightheaded and had to catch my breath to regain my composure.

After the procedure, the nurse instructed me to get dressed and said she would call me at home in a few days with the pathology results. I left the clinic still in shock, trying to comprehend what was happening.

When Michael arrived home, I was an emotional wreck. I had been crying all evening. Once I explained my mammogram results, he embraced me and said, "Everything will be okay, and we'll get through this together." We were both praying for a miracle.

Several days passed before Dr. Osmont's nurse called. She said Michael and I needed to meet with Dr. Osmont the next day to discuss my pathology report. After our conversation, all I could think about was dying from breast cancer. This scenario was not supposed to be happening, because my mammograms from the previous years had always been negative for breast cancer. Where had the cancer been concealing itself until now?

The next day, we met with Dr. Osmont. He explained he needed to perform a tissue biopsy to gain better knowledge and determine the stage of cancer involved. The procedure was considered outpatient surgery and had to be performed the next morning. Before we left the hospital, we completed the necessary paperwork authorizing the tissue biopsy. We wanted to make sure everything would go as smoothly as possible.

The following morning, I registered for surgery, not knowing what the prognosis would be. I prayed for the strength to be able to handle the situation regardless of the stage of breast cancer. Shortly after registering, I was taken to my room. My mother-in-law, Dolores, sister-in-law Valerie, and cousin Betty Mae met us at the hospital for prayer and support. Everyone prayed the cancer had been detected early for my well-being.

The surgical team arrived ten minutes later, introduced themselves, and took me to the operating room. The surgery took an hour. After surgery, I was taken to recovery, where I remained until being discharged.

Mentally, I was not prepared for this disruption in my life. Now I was dealing with the possibility of closing the deli, which had only been open for seven months and was doing well. We had also established a lunch clientele and had worked diligently to build the business. Now I was faced with the possibility of seeing my dreams vanish before my very eyes. I prayed for God to intervene in my life and to resolve the situation I faced.

Several days later we met with Dr. Osmont, and he explained the breast cancer was an aggressive form due to my positive estrogen receptors. Breast cancer cells thrive on estrogen. Dr. Osmont's strategy for treating the cancer was to perform a radical mastectomy on the right breast. He recommended the surgery be performed within the next ten days to prevent the spreading of the cancer.

We went home and prayed for God to heal my body of breast cancer. We also prayed the cancer had been detected early enough to increase my chances of surviving this deadly disease. We needed to notify our families with the disappointing news. My mother needed to make arrangements to take time off from work. I also reminded her of those flannel pajamas I had requested during our visit in January. I also decided to take the entire ten days to mentally prepare myself for the closing of the deli and allow time for my mother to make arrangements to fly to Mobile.

My mother arrived the day before the surgery. Michael and I met her at the airport. I was relieved when she stepped off the plane. I knew everything would be all right. Regardless of how old we are, in desperate times we always want our mothers around. And she was a blessing to have with us during this critical time in our lives.

My mother is a remarkable woman; whenever there is need for her nurturing and love, we can depend on her to be there. She will travel across the country to support her family during any crisis that may occur. She is always willing to provide her love and support.

Later that night, the three of us went out to dinner, but we returned home early to prepare ourselves emotionally for surgery in the morning.

Before going to sleep that night, I prayed to God to wake me thirty minutes after surgery. I so desperately wanted this nightmare to end. However, when morning arrived, I had not slept well; throughout the night I had continued to experience anxiety attacks. They left me feeling anxious, so we left the house earlier than planned to register for surgery. My in-laws were meeting us at the hospital for moral support and prayer.

Michael, my mother, and I arrived at the hospital at 6:00 a.m. I was immediately taken to the waiting area, and I remained there until surgery. My curiosity wanted to know who was assisting with my surgery; therefore, I requested to meet with everyone on the team.

After all, I was putting my life into the hands of strangers. On the way to surgery, I asked the anesthesiologist how long I would be unconscious.

He replied, "Quite some time," and proceeded to put the oxygen mask over my face.

I removed the mask and informed him I would only be unconscious for a short time. The anesthesiologist and the team continued to roll my bed down the hallway toward the operating room and began to laugh. The anesthesiologist again returned the mask to my face, only to have me remove it again. I replied by telling them I would only be unconscious for a brief time. The team finally stopped rolling the bed and asked what made me think that. My response was, "I had asked God to wake me thirty minutes after surgery, and He promised He would." That is the last thing I remember before waking up.

I remember waking up in recovery, feeling as if I was dreaming; everything appeared cloudy. The first object I focused on was an enormous clock hanging on the wall. If my calculations were correct, I had awakened forty minutes after surgery. God kept His promise.

As the anesthesia began to wear off, I discovered I did not have any sensation in my right arm. To my left I noticed four nurses sitting around a table, playing cards. I called out for their assistance in a very low voice, only to be ignored. I waited a few minutes and called out to them again and was stilled ignored. A couple of minutes later, on my third call, Michael apparently heard my voice and came to my rescue. I explained the situation regarding my arm and asked him to rub it to get the circulation going.

Well, there was finally a response from one of the nurses. She said Michael should not rub my arm, because it could cause a blood clot. If they had responded to my earlier calls, this entire situation could have been avoided. Instead, I felt they were being rude and ignoring my cries for help. Shortly after that situation, a male orderly took me to my private room.

Upon arriving at my room, I was surprised to discover many floral arrangements had been delivered. One of them was a beautiful arrangement from my favorite cousin, Tyrone, who is in the military. I was delighted to see so many people cared enough about my well-being to take the time to send flowers. That touched my heart. It's during times of despair when we learn who our real friends and loved ones are.

Once I was settled, Michael, my mother, and my in-laws came to visit. I was pleased to see them but was exhausted, and therefore I requested they leave. Dr. Osmont entered the room a few minutes later and asked how I was doing. I inquired as to how long I would be hospitalized. He replied, "Two to three days."

After our discussion I tried to get some sleep and failed. Each time I dozed off, there was a nurse poking me and asking me questions. I informed her that I just wanted to get some sleep. One of the nurses smiled and said, "Good luck."

It was now dinnertime. I thought this would be the perfect opportunity to steal a nap while the other patients were having their meals. But no such luck. Immediately following dinner, it was the same routine all over again. Every hour, on the hour, a nurse checked on me. After nine o'clock the knocks did not come so frequently.

Several hours passed without a visit from the nurses, and then there was a knock at the door. The nurse needed to take my vital signs. She asked if I was experiencing any discomfort or having any pain. I informed her I was having a difficult time trying to sleep. She suggested I use the PC (pain control) machine.

Apparently there was a puzzling look on my face, and she realized I did not have a clue as to what she was referring to. She pointed to the machine on the floor, which had an IV leading to my arm, and told me the PC machine held morphine, which would assist me with sleeping.

She instructed me on how to use the machine and demonstrated how to press the button a few times to release the medication. At that time I was desperate and willing to try anything to get some sleep.

Between the morphine and using the bedpan, I had a difficult night. I prayed for morning to come; my body was exhausted. Around 2:00 a.m., a male nurse entered my room to take my vital signs. He drew blood from my right arm, the side on which the mastectomy had been performed. Several minutes later, his supervisor entered the room to evaluate his performance, and she panicked when she realized he had drawn blood from my right arm. She began screaming that he wasn't supposed to draw blood from the arm on the side where the mastectomy had been performed. She then explained that during surgery the doctor had removed eighteen lymph nodes from underneath my arm. Lymph nodes help fight off infections. Without lymph nodes, I was at risk of contracting an infection.

The nurse explained the consequence of not letting anyone draw blood or take vital signs from my right arm for the next five years.

She left the room, only to return a few minutes later with a sign she had made, which she posted above my bed. The sign read, "Please do not take vitals from patient's right arm due to mastectomy."

After the confusion, I tried to get some sleep, but it was pointless. The IV saline solution continued to pass straight through me. I was compelled to use the bedpan throughout the night. This was my first experience using a bedpan, and I prayed it was the last.

Morning finally arrived, and two nurse's aides entered my room.

We talked briefly, and I began to sit up and get out of bed. They both questioned me; they wanted to know what I was doing. I explained I was going to the bathroom. They wanted to know who had authorized this privilege. I lied and said my doctor had given me permission. They both said, "You are telling a lie," because none of the doctors had made their morning rounds. I mentioned I did not care and was going to the bathroom anyway. On that note, I proceeded to get out of bed, and when my feet hit the floor, that's when all hell broke loose.

The IV solution ran straight through me, and I began to urinate on the floor. The two nurse's aides laughed as I begged them for their assistance. One of the aides finally pushed a trashcan underneath me to catch the remainder of urine. That was an embarrassing moment!

As I lay in bed, contemplating my next move without having an accident, the light bulb came on in my head. Determined not to use the bedpan, I continued to analyze the situation. The two obstacles preventing me from executing a successful move were the PC machine and the IV cart. I knew I had to lose one of the carts, so I transferred the IV bag to the PC cart, making it easier for me to maneuver. Once they were consolidated, I pushed the IV cart against the wall.

Now the opportunity had arrived to execute the plan. Would it be successful, or would it fail? I just barely made it. I knew next time my actions needed to be more rapid. On my next visit to the bathroom, I planned to have plenty of time to spare, but only time would tell.

Later that morning, a nurse entered the room to check my vital signs and noticed the IV cart against the wall; she panicked, not giving me the opportunity to explain the consolidation of the carts.

After she checked my vital signs, she left the room, shaking her head and mumbling to herself. When Dr. Osmont's assistant, Dr. Byrd, entered my room, he stated the nurses had said I was being difficult.

He wanted to order lab work, and if it proved to be good he would discharge me that day. I was ecstatic; surgery had taken place less than twenty-four hours ago, and there was an outstanding possibility of me being discharged. I impatiently waited for Michael's arrival to share the wonderful news.

When Michael entered the room, the first words out of my mouth were, "I'm being discharged." Well, he thought I had lost my mind until I explained Dr. Byrd's decision regarding the lab work. I explained that if my lab work was fine I would be discharged, so we both waited for the results to come back.

Dr. Byrd received the lab results around noon, and they were excellent, so he discharged me. I began to get dressed while Michael completed the discharge paperwork. Once dressed, I decided to give several floral arrangements to patients. When Michael returned, I was dressed and ready to go. The nurse was ready as well, and she wheeled me to the door. If I did not know any better, I would have thought she was trying to get rid of me!

When we arrived home, I was exhausted and wanted to sleep, but first I needed to see my incision. As Michael began to carefully unwrap the bandages, I wasn't sure if I could handle what was about to be revealed. Once the final bandage was removed, I realized my body was disfigured and would be so for the rest of my life. I wondered if I could adjust to this drastic change in my appearance. One day I had two breasts, and the next I had only one, with an empty space and a scar where the other breast had been.

There were plenty of staples and stitches holding my incision together, along with two Jackson-Pratt drainage bottles on each side of my waist. The incision extended from my right armpit to the middle of my chest. I asked Michael if he still loved me with only one breast. He said yes and began to rewrap my incision, and he assisted me into my flannel pajamas. The warm, plush feeling of the flannel pajamas comforted my entire body.

As I prepared for bed, the telephone began to ring. My family and friends were calling to see how my surgery had gone. I would hear my mother say, "She's home. Would you like to speak with her?" Everyone I spoke with was amazed and wanted to know how I had managed to be released from the hospital so soon. I mentioned the nurses said I was being difficult and wasn't following my doctor's orders.

Later that evening my friends Helen and Diane stopped by for a visit. They wanted to see how my recovery was coming along. Helen wanted to know if it was all right for her to view my mastectomy.

She was curious as to what a mastectomy involved; just in case she might be confronted with one. They both wanted to know if my body felt different. As strange as it may sound, the only discomfort I had was in my arm; otherwise, it felt as if I still had both breasts.

Several days later, I continued to receive plenty of telephone calls from loved ones regarding my recovery. I was feeling fantastic and had taken the initiative to start my therapy of "walking the wall." "Walking the wall" is an exercise in which I extend my arm up against the wall as high as it can reach and repeat the motion as often as possible. This exercise eliminates the chances of developing a condition called *cold shoulder*. The condition could have developed as a result of the removal of the lymph nodes from underneath my armpit. Some women develop cold shoulder as a result of a lack of arm movement.

It's better to bite the bullet in the beginning and deal with the pain from the exercise than to lose a lifetime of mobility.

I refused to let the breast cancer affect me. I never missed a beat.

I was vibrant and full of life. After all, I had my entire life ahead of me, and I planned to enjoy every moment. My loved ones were there to see me through this difficult chapter in my life.

After two weeks of recovery I was doing fantastic. My mother and I agreed she should return home. She called the airline and changed her reservation to an earlier flight for the following morning. My mother, Michael, and I decided to go out to dinner to celebrate my recovery. We returned early so she could prepare for her departure. That night, before going to bed, I thanked God for his blessings and asked him to take care of my mother on her journey home. I must admit I was going to miss her, but I was capable of caring for myself.

The next morning, Michael took my mother to the airport. While Michael was gone, I had too much idle time on my hands. My mind could not relax. The deli had been closed for several weeks, and I wasn't functioning 100%. I prayed my clientele would return once the deli reopened; we had worked diligently to build the business.

When the deli closed, I posted a sign stating we would be closed for two weeks, but now it was entering the third week and I had no idea when I would be returning. And I was also thinking about our 1997 family reunion, which Michael and I were sponsoring in July. I hoped things would go as scheduled, because I had planned for us to have a spectacular weekend. There would be an award ceremony in which the family members would be acknowledged for their achievements over the past two years.

There were achievement awards to write and gifts to be purchased for presentations during the ceremony. There was enough work to keep me occupied for several months; therefore, I needed to recover as quickly as possible.

Chapter Two:

Chemotherapy

THREE WEEKS PASSED AND IT was time for my follow-up for the mastectomy. I signed in while Michael located seats for us. We sat patiently and waited for my name to be called. When I was called, the nurse escorted us to the examining room and instructed me to get undressed. I undressed and changed into a gown. Michael and I spoke briefly to pass the time as we waited for Dr. Osmont.

Dr. Osmont and his nurse entered the room. He asked how my recovery was coming along. I told him it was going well but that I was anxious to have the stitches and staples removed, along with the two drainage bottles. My reasoning was that I needed to get back to the deli and recover my lost business. Having the drainage bottles presented limitations, making it difficult for me to move around.

Dr. Osmont examined my incision and said it was healing beautifully. Therefore, he went ahead and removed the stitches and staples. Another appointment was scheduled in one week for the removal of the drainage bottles; at that time Dr. Osmont would discuss the possibility of me returning to work. My returning to the deli depended upon the mastectomy healing on schedule. The healing process was critical and needed to be monitored carefully; this would help me avoid any setbacks or complications. The anticipation of returning to work was awesome, and I waited eagerly for my next appointment.

We returned to the clinic the following week to have the drainage bottles removed. I thought the removing of the drainage bottles was going to be a breeze. Boy was I wrong! When Dr. Osmont began to remove the tube from the first drainage bottle, I became speechless. As he began to pull the drainage bottle, it felt as if my body was on fire. The tube ripped through my body, causing my flesh to burn like an inferno.

Michael was holding my hand and reassuring me the procedure would be over soon. Well, I screamed "Jesus, God, and Glory!" and bit Michael's hand. I screamed and told the three of them to get away from me. Nothing could have prepared me for the intense pain I was experiencing.

Laying there in shock, still in disbelief. I had no idea removing the drainage bottles would cause such excruciating pain. There was about sixteen inches of tubing inside of me, and my flesh had grown attached to the tube and had become one with it. Finally, the nurse said, "Now, Brenda, the doctor needs to remove the other drainage bottle."

When he began to remove the second drainage bottle, I said those words again, "Jesus, God, Glory!" and bit Michael once more.

Again I told them to get away from me. I lay there trying to regain my composure and prepare myself to go home.

After everything was over, Michael and I had a good laugh. I dressed and scheduled my next appointment. Even though I laughed afterwards, I will always remember the pain I experienced from the removal of the drainage bottles. I hope I never experience that intense pain again.

At my next appointment, Dr. Osmont did not allow me to return to work. He felt it was too soon. My heart was filled with disappointment. He said that we would discuss chemotherapy at the next appointment. Dr. Osmont recommended Dr. Mann from Cross Hospital. He is considered one of the top oncologists in the field. Dr. Mann has been practicing chemotherapy in Chicago since the late 1950s.

On the day of my first chemotherapy session, I decided to go alone. I assumed that since the mastectomy was such a breeze, chemotherapy would be as well. I knew it would be difficult getting the injections, because of my phobia of needles, but, I was willing to go forward. When I arrived at the oncology office, I signed in, filled out the forms, and waited to be called. The waiting area was decorated beautifully and had an inviting atmosphere. There were plenty of magazines to read. The staff was very accommodating, making sure my needs were met.

The nurse called me and escorted me to an examining room. She said Dr. Mann would be with me shortly. I undressed and put on a gown and read several magazines while waiting. When he arrived, I saw he was much older than I had anticipated. He was in his early 70's, but he appeared to be full of life and had an exceptional sense of humor. He introduced himself and examined my mastectomy to make sure my incision had healed. He said that everything looked fine and that I could start treatments right away. Dr. Mann explained his oncology nurse would be administering the treatments. She explained the procedure in detail; it would take an hour to complete and consist of two injections delivered intravenously into my hand.

The rooms in which the chemo treatments are given were comfortable and painted different shades of blue. Each room contained a large recliner and had a color television mounted on the wall. The nurse began the procedure by inserting an IV into my arm. I wanted to cry but fought back the tears. I had promised myself I would be strong and would embrace the first injection of chemotherapy. I watched as she pushed those chemicals into my veins. I could see the orange solution as it began to circulate through my veins. Oh Lord, I could have passed out.

Never once had I imagined anything like this in my wildest dreams. All I could do was wonder what the hell was going on. The chemotherapy was horrible, and it began to burn my skin. I wanted to leave after the first injection but stayed for the second, wondering if I could make it through the session. I began to pray and ask God to give me the strength to continue. I realized I wasn't prepared for the chemotherapy procedure; I had no idea what the sessions would entail.

In my mind, I believed it was morally wrong and inhumane to have toxic chemicals injected into my veins. I wondered what good could possibly come from these treatments. I wanted everything to end as quickly as possible. By that time I could even smell the chemicals coming out of my pores and could taste them in my mouth. As the taste became stronger, I became ill. Once the treatments were over, I sat there trying to comprehend what I had just endured. I found my way to the front desk and scheduled another appointment.

This was the first time since my mastectomy I had experienced depression. I walked to my car in a daze, wondering how anyone could sit and have poisonous chemicals injected into their veins. My mind couldn't comprehend the significance of the treatment I had just received. In order to kill cancer cells, healthy cells in my body would die as well. Therefore, I knew that by the time the chemotherapy sessions were completed, every cell in my body would be affected in some way.

On my way home, the sicknesses worsened. Several times I had to pull over to vomit. I never once fathomed the therapy would cause me to become ill so quickly. Nothing could have prepared me for the side effects I was to encounter.

When Michael arrived home, he knew immediately I wasn't feeling well. I explained I had been vomiting all day. He went to the store to purchase ginger ale sodas. When he returned, I prayed the soda would provide relief. I remained ill throughout the night, and it left Michael feeling helpless; there wasn't anything he could do to eliminate my discomfort.

Finally, daylight arrived. I had stopped vomiting, and I tried to get some sleep. Michael wanted to stay home, but I assured him I would be all right. He promised to call me throughout the day. All morning I tried to eat but couldn't keep any food down. I felt as if I was dying, and I had no clue of how to improve the situation. All I understood was that my body was being destroyed by toxic chemicals, and I wondered how such a radical treatment could have a positive ending.

When Michael arrived home, he prepared homemade chicken soup and cornbread. I barely had an appetite. All I wanted to do was to sleep the night away and pray the following morning would be better. I never imagined having treatments to save my life would have me feeling deathly ill. Later that night, while feeling terrible, I wondered how I would complete another session. I found myself asking God to give me the strength to continue. The thought of returning to the hospital and willingly allowing poisonous chemicals to be injected into my veins seemed impossible.

On the third day after chemotherapy, I received a call from the oncology nurse. She wanted to know my status. I informed her I felt as if I was dying. She asked why no one had notified them regarding my condition. I explained that while in the waiting area I had read an article which stated people going through chemotherapy often believe they are dying because of the sickness associated with the treatments. The nurse also mentioned there were medications to prevent nausea and anxiety. She stated I could pick up the prescriptions and have them filled at the pharmacy before my next appointment.

I picked up the prescriptions and headed to the pharmacy. Once I had arrived at the pharmacy, I was appalled at the outrageous cost of the medications. One of the prescriptions wasn't covered under my insurance. I was shocked to find out how expensive the medication was. The medication to prevent nausea cost $1,000. I remember wondering how the government could allow citizens to pay an exorbitant cost for medication to avoid becoming ill as a result of medical treatments. Needless to say, I left the pharmacy without the medication.

Thank goodness Michael had retired from the army several years ago and had medical benefits. When I arrived home, I immediately contacted Keesler Air Force Base in Biloxi, Mississippi to see if they carried the medication. I was relieved to learn the pharmacy carried the medication.

Biloxi is only one hour away, and I find the drive always relaxes me; I enjoy just watching the trees as I pass them by.

While at the air force base, I decided to do some shopping at the post exchange until the prescription was filled. When I returned to the pharmacy, I was surprised to find the prescription had not been filled. The pharmacist needed to get authorization from the post commander to dispense fifty pills because of the exorbitant cost. I had to wait until the post commander notified the pharmacist. Finally, the authorization was given, and even then I was only given nine pills. I would need to return every three weeks for my refills. I recall wondering how our government allows such outrageous prices for medications.

Weeks had passed since my chemotherapy session, and I was still sick; no one could have prepared me for the lengthy side effects associated with the injections. Several times I had even wondered if death would be more comforting. My mind was always filled with depressing thoughts. In such a short time, I had developed sensitivity to the sunlight and was constantly feeling exhausted; even my taste buds had been affected.

I was also wrestling with the thoughts of not being able to reopen the deli. I knew for certain my clientele was lost, and it would be almost impossible to recover the business. My life was spinning out of control. These unplanned events were unfolding right before my eyes. All I could think about was my dreams coming to an end. At that moment I wished I could change the scenario, but I knew it was impossible.

One day while lying in bed, thinking about the direction my life had taken, I received a phone call from our pastor. He and one of the deacons were having a difficult time trying to locate our townhouse. Thank goodness they called; it allowed me the opportunity to change into an African garment which was more appropriate for greeting guests. When they arrived, we had prayer, and as they were leaving, the pastor handed me an envelope.

After closing the door, I opened the envelope, and found, to my surprise, that the church had taken up a collection for us. I was extremely touched by their generosity and kindness.

The weeks passed quickly, and it was time for another chemotherapy session; once again I decided to go alone. Before leaving home I took the nausea and anxiety medications and felt everything would go well. I also took slices of lemon and peppermint candy to rid me of the disgusting aftertaste from the chemotherapy.

I signed in and took a seat and waited to be called. To my surprise, the nurse was prepared, and we immediately started. I sat there and watched in amazement as she pushed the IV into my hand. Once the IV was in, she began slowly to release the chemo into my veins. I watched as it appeared in a circular form in my hand.

During the session, I requested that the nurse stop several times; she finally asked if there was someone I could call for moral support. I answered no, so she proceeded with the treatment as I cried the entire time. Regardless of how many patients she had given chemotherapy, she could never imagine the anxiety I was experiencing unless she had experienced it herself.

Finally the session ended, but it took thirty minutes longer than it should have to administer the injections because of my interrupting her several times.

After gaining my composure, I left the hospital. On the way home, I became ill. The medication for the nausea provided no relief. After pulling over several times, I wondered how I would make it home. All I could do was pray and ask God for the strength to arrive safely.

After arriving home, I immediately undressed, prepared some soup, and went straight to bed. I felt dreadful and was contemplating not returning to the hospital for the remaining treatments. I had several weeks to ponder my decision.

I finally dozed off, and when I awakened, Michael was home; I was relieved to see him. I knew I was in excellent hands. He wanted to know if he could do anything to comfort me. I told him just his being there was enough.

The following morning, I felt well enough to work on the family reunion ceremony. Luckily, I had already booked the hotel and banquet. I had started writing the achievement awards; I wanted everything to be spectacular! I was determined not to let the chemotherapy dictate my life. Somehow I was going to overcome it. For a few hours that day, I was able to work on the awards. Every so often, I would develop hot flashes that lasted five minutes or more. This caused me to take several breaks to cool off. At times it felt as if my body temperature was over 100 degrees. No one had prepared me for the hot flashes I was experiencing.

By then my hair was falling out, and I decided it was time to purchase a wig, along with plenty of popsicles to gain relief from the hot flashes, although I soon learned the hot flashes worsened while wearing the wig. Sometimes while driving I would experience hot flashes and remove my wig; then I would notice the driver in the vehicle next to mine with an alarmed expression on his or her face.

The hot flashes were so unbearable that I called my friend Helen, who is a hair stylist, and asked her if she could shave my head. She agreed, so I drove to her house. When I left, I was completely bald, and was stunning with my beautiful bald head, which represented life.

Although my head was shaved, the hot flashes continued. Upon my arriving home, I undressed, took a shower, and ate plenty of popsicles, hoping for some relief. My body finally began to cool down, but I couldn't help but wonder what other side effects I would encounter. I knew things were only going to get worse. After my body temperature returned to normal, I continued to work on the awards for the ceremony. After all, I had nothing but time on my hands.

Even though I had the energy to work on the family reunion, I was still unable to reopen the deli because of the many side effects I was constantly experiencing. The hot flashes became a normal part of my life, and my body was out of alignment. My taste buds had been destroyed by the chemotherapy. I had not anticipated this change.

The only foods I could tolerate were chicken noodle soup, mustard and turnip greens, tomatoes, and cornbread. I ate this for breakfast, lunch and dinner. The only two beverages I tolerated were water and ginger ale. Worst of all, I hated the smell of fried chicken, which happens to be Michael's favorite dish. When he fried chicken, he tried his best to accommodate me by closing the bedroom door. I was devastated as to how the chemotherapy was affecting my entire body.

Three weeks later, it was time for another chemotherapy session; as I drove, I began to experience anxiety attacks. As I neared the hospital, I turned my car around and headed back home. My thoughts were, *There is no way I'm going to the hospital to subject myself to another treatment. I* began to cry uncontrollably, but I knew the proper thing to do was turn around and continue in the direction of the hospital.

When I arrived, it was obvious I was upset. Both the doctor and the nurse tried to comfort me. But it was pointless; I began to stress even more. The nurse finally asked if there was someone who could come and sit with me. I immediately thought of Helen, since it was her day off.

I called Helen and explained the situation, and she agreed to come. The nurse and I waited for Helen's arrival before continuing with the injections. We both were relieved when we saw Helen walk through the door. Although Helen was there, it was pointless. I cried the entire time as she held my hand for moral support. After the session ended, we left the hospital. She followed me home to make sure I arrived safely.

Lying in bed, I wondered again if there was an alternative cancer treatment to increase my chances of survival without having poisonous chemicals injected into my body. I still believed that if the cancer did not kill me, the chemotherapy would. And if I was going to die, I wanted to be remembered as the "Energizer lady," as Michael calls me. There was no way I was going to have a depressing funeral service at which I received pity due to my suffering. I wanted my loved ones to celebrate my homecoming and play my favorite Gospel CD to finalize my earthly departure.

By then I had come to terms regarding my business, and I eventually decided to close the deli. My decision was a difficult one to make, but I could not continue paying rent and utilities on a business that wasn't turning a profit. I came to the realization that selling the restaurant equipment would be the logical thing to do. I contacted the wholesale warehouse regarding buying back some of the items. Once I explained my situation, they agreed to buy back the items as long as they were in excellent condition.

Next I had to sell the appliances and try to get a reasonable price.

I needed to rent a truck to transport the other items to the resale shop. I checked with the owner to see if I could sell the tables and chairs. I had to accept his offer, regardless of the financial loss. I had been without an income for four months and was feeling desperate. I hated facing the reality of my dreams coming to an end, but I saw no other alternative.

Once I made the arrangements regarding the closing of the restaurant, it was time to focus on our family reunion. I was grateful I had planned the picnic to be in our backyard. The backyard is beautiful and spacious, and it has a play area for the children. I had even taken into consideration the seniors that were participating in the reunion. In our family we have numerous seniors who are in their late 80s and 90s.

The temperatures in Mobile during the summer months are extremely warm and can reach the high 90s before noon. I had also considered my situation regarding my lupus: the sun and heat are my worst enemies. When my body temperature increases as a result of the heat, I become ill. And if that occurs, I can end up in bed for several days or weeks.

Helen picked me up for my next chemotherapy session. I told myself I wasn't going to stress out and would tolerate the treatments. I prayed on the matter and asked God to give me the strength to get through the session. I felt that with Helen's presence I would do well. As we neared the hospital, I began to have a panic attack and requested that she take me back home. She did as I requested and headed back in the direction of my house, but she explained the consequences of not completing the treatments. All I could do was cry, because I knew she was right. I began to pray for the strength to continue with the treatments. At that moment I wished chemotherapy could have been administered orally in a pill. That would have been terrific and psychologically easier.

When we arrived at the oncology office, the nurse was prepared and was thrilled to see Helen. She thought this session would go smoothly, and I prayed the same. But once I saw the IV and the two injections on the table, I began to panic. I cried the entire time as Helen held my hand. I ate lemon slices and peppermint candy to eliminate the unpleasant taste in my mouth. I appeared to have more difficulties with chemotherapy than most people. I wasn't sure if it was because of the lupus, my phobia of needles, or just the chemotherapy itself. I understood the importance of the chemotherapy; I just refused to accept the knowledge of killing healthy cells. And as a result of the many difficulties I experienced from the chemotherapy, I decided not to return to the hospital for my final session.

A month had passed since my last session, and I felt exceptionally well. I had planned a birthday party for Michael; our family and friends were to bring the food on Sunday for the celebration after church. I was looking forward to this festive occasion after months of despair.

When Sunday arrived, I had to literally force myself out of bed.

Although I was weak and exhausted, it wasn't going to prevent me from celebrating Michael's birthday. The guests began to arrive just as I prepared to get dressed.

There was plenty of food and cake. The day was beautiful, and everyone was having a terrific time. Michael received an abundance of birthday cards and gifts. The party was going well, and then there was a knock at the door. When I answered the door, to my surprise, there stood a postman; he had a registered letter that required my signature. I signed for the letter. When I opened the envelope, I saw it was from Dr. Mann. The letter stated that if I did not complete chemotherapy, no doctor in the state of Alabama would consent in treating me.

I handed Michael the letter to read, and we both decided not to let the news spoil his birthday celebration.

After the party ended, Michael and I had a conversation regarding the completion of chemotherapy. We agreed I should call the hospital Monday and have someone explain the meaning of the letter. I felt it should have been my decision to complete or not complete treatments. After all, it was my life and my body. I was totally unaware I needed my doctor's consent to end chemotherapy.

On Monday morning I called Dr. Mann's office and spoke with the nurse. She explained that because I had begun chemotherapy, the doctor was responsible for my well-being. She mentioned that if I died, my family could file a malpractice suit against the hospital and the doctor. I then understood the significance of the letter and decided the appropriate thing to do was complete the last session.

Who could blame the oncologist and the hospital for covering themselves? I'm sure I would have made the same decision under those circumstances.

I knew it would be a difficult session, but it had to be done. I made the appointment for the following week, allowing myself time to prepare emotionally for the final chemotherapy session.

My last chemotherapy session was the most difficult one. Helen was unable to accompany me to the hospital for various reasons. My anxiety level was extremely high before I left home. When I arrived at the oncology office, I signed in and went straight to the restroom. Several nurses finally had to retrieve me as I cried the entire time. Regardless of what the nurses and the doctor said or did, nothing comforted me. After the chemotherapy injection, Dr. Mann requested a blood test to check my white blood count. I refused to allow the nurse to prick my finger. I figured that since this was the last session, there was no reason for the blood test. I knew in my heart I would never be returning to the hospital again. As I drove out of the hospital parking lot, I never looked back; that chapter of my life was over.

This time when I drove home and became ill, I was relieved by the situation, because this was the last time I would travel that road. I called Michael from my cell phone and informed him of the wonderful news that I had completed chemotherapy. When I arrived home, I did my normal routine, had soup, and went straight to bed. I knew that when I awakened, this nightmare would finally be behind me, and I was looking forward to the beginning of a new day.

To my surprise, I found when I awakened that I had broken out with shingles that resembled a rash on the back of my left leg. I'm sure they developed as a result of my being so terribly stressed out. I accepted the condition because I was finally finished with chemotherapy.

Later that evening I called my mother and shared my exciting news regarding my completion of therapy. She was consumed with joy, and she could finally have peace of mind.

Chapter Three:

Taking Control

Now that chemotherapy was behind me, I could focus my attention on the family reunion. The reunion was in two weeks, and I still had floral arrangements to design and achievement awards to write. I had confirmed the banquet and secured the tent, tables, and chairs for the picnic. I was relieved everything was coming together as planned. Michael and I were hosting a welcoming dinner for our family members arriving on Friday. They would be greeted with a feast fit for kings and queens. I hoped everyone would be bringing his or her appetite, because there would be plenty of delectable foods to satisfy every appetite.

We purchased the food on Wednesday to ensure we had everything required for a successful event. Michael had begun preparing for Saturday's barbeque. There were plenty of ribs and chicken that needed to be grilled. I prepared a variety of dishes and baked an enormous homemade peach cobbler.

The anticipation of seeing our relatives was electrifying. We had worked diligently for this event and planned for everyone to have a fantastic time. After dinner, Michael and some of the family members were planning to go to Biloxi, Mississippi to the casinos for entertainment. I would take the opportunity to relax and prepare for Saturday's picnic.

On Friday we had an excellent turnout. Two years had passed since our last reunion, and we were excited to see one another. I received many compliments regarding how beautiful I was with my stunning bald head. I must admit to myself that my bald head enhanced my appearance. I never mentioned to our family that my baldness was the result of chemotherapy treatments, along with Helen's excellent barber skills.

After dinner, everyone was ready for some excitement and entertainment. They all gathered themselves together to line up for the convoy. Michael was the leader; he ensured everyone knew the way. I remained home and continued to prepare for the picnic. After I finished, I decided to turn in early so I could be rejuvenated for Saturday morning.

Michael and some of the family members returned early Saturday morning. I wondered how he would manage without any sleep. He and Cousin Joe had planned to barbeque together, but the plan was spoiled when Joe fell asleep, leaving Michael alone to man the grill.

Luckily, Uncle Clinton arrived that morning: he was a welcome sight with his cowboy hat and boots. Uncle Clinton is my mother's older living brother who lives in Houston, Texas.

I started to prepare the picnic area. I needed to work quickly to avoid the extreme heat and sun. Decorating the area would take an hour, and I wanted everything to be perfect, right down to the centerpiece on each table. The weather was beautiful; the humidity was low. I only wished it could remain that way for the remainder of the day. The Weather Channel had forecast afternoon showers, but I hoped they would be proven wrong.

The family members began arriving around 10:00 a.m. Everything was prepared and ready to go. As the family members arrived, I handed out the T-shirts. These were not typical family reunion T-shirts: they were available with four different African themes and three colors to choose from. I chose these particular T-shirts because they could be worn at another casual gathering with a favorite pair of jeans.

I remained in the house throughout the day, avoiding the heat. The senior family members chose to remain outside but had the option to retreat into the house if necessary. As for me, I worked the picnic from the back door, giving orders and making sure everything remained organized and ran smoothly. Around 1:00 p.m., it began to rain, but no one was affected, because we had the tent.

July is a rainy month in Alabama because of hurricane season; therefore I knew we needed to be prepared for the weather. I was ecstatic that the weather did not interfere with the event. The family members never missed a beat. They had a marvelous time socializing and enjoying delicious foods and festivities. My only regret was that I was unable to participate.

The picnic ended at 3:00 p.m., and everyone went back to the hotel for some relaxation. The banquet would take place at the hotel at 7:00 p.m that night. Michael and I remained home; we both needed our rest. The hotel was only five minutes away, so we had plenty of time to rest, get dressed, and arrive on time.

The award ceremony would be a total surprise to everyone. When I mailed the information regarding the reunion, I requested everyone wear formal dress attire for the banquet. I wanted the banquet to have a formal atmosphere and be an unforgettable occasion

Michael was dressed in his dinner tuxedo, and I was wearing a navy gown with a beautiful beaded jacket. Everyone was dressed as I had requested. We appeared as though we were at the Academy Awards and it was being televised nationwide. I was delighted the agenda was going as planned.

My appearance had changed dramatically for the banquet: I was wearing a stylish wig which complemented my appearance. As the family members arrived, Michael and I greeted our guests and thanked them for attending the 1997 Simpson, Scott, and Brim Family Reunion. We expressed our gratitude for their participation at this memorable occasion. I made a special announcement for the family members who had supported me during my bout with breast cancer and chemotherapy. Other family members were flabbergasted to learn I had breast cancer. That's when I explained the reason for my bald head. Many people had thought it was a fashion statement. We all had a hearty laugh then we explained the agenda for the evening.

The Achievement Award ceremony acknowledged our family members' successes and accomplishments over the last two years.

There were several categories, including an Acknowledgement Award for my sister Kimberly, who had graduated from Chicago State University with honors. My cousin Gloria received an award for her accomplishments in the military as a commissioned officer.

There was an award for positive male role model, and for dedicated military soldiers, past and present. There was an award for the oldest family member and awards for the entire graduating class of 1997.

Some family members received everlasting floral arrangements for their achievements. I presented my mother with a crystal hourglass, which represented the time she spent with me during my recovery. Everyone who received an award was elated.

After the ceremony, we had dinner and danced the night away. I was enthralled. We had a spectacular evening. The banquet ended at 11 p.m., and we made the announcement that everyone was invited to our home for Sunday breakfast. Michael and I continued to entertain in the lobby, but around midnight we said goodnight and headed home. We needed to rise early to prepare breakfast for seventy-five to eighty people.

I wanted breakfast to be delicious as well as unforgettable. I planned a luscious eight-course meal. I looked forward to preparing our last meal together. I get satisfaction out of knowing people are enjoying food I have prepared. Delicious food always brings out the best in people.

On Sunday morning, everyone began arriving for breakfast. We knew this would be the last time some of us would see or speak to each other until the next reunion, which was scheduled to take place in Houston in 1999.

There was a large assortment of foods to please everyone's appetite. We all had a marvelous time hugging each other and saying our goodbyes. Some of the men stayed behind to assist Michael with taking down the tent, tables, and chairs. I started organizing the house while we still had plenty of assistance. We finished organizing the house and yard later that afternoon. We were overjoyed that the reunion was successful, and we knew it would be etched in everyone's memories for years to come. I did not know about Michael, but I was looking forward to sponsoring another reunion.

It had been six months since my life had changed and now that the reunion, breast cancer, and chemotherapy were behind me, I decided to do some traveling. Helen was off work as a result of foot surgery; designating her as my perfect companion. The anticipation of being on the highway, marveling at God's creations, was awesome.

"Our first trip will be to Chicago," I said to her.

We arrived in Chicago on Friday evening. Being home in the Windy City felt fantastic. During our visit, we stayed with my father on the south side. We settled in early for the night to be well rested for our adventure in the morning. We had a cookout planned for Saturday afternoon; this allowed my friends and family an opportunity to stop by and socialize.

On Saturday morning, Helen was astonished at the enormous size of the city and also at how many people reside in the metropolitan area. The weather was cool, which is typical for Chicago during autumn. The leaves had already begun to change colors and fall from the trees. I adore the various colors of leaves associated with the season. Autumn has always been my favorite season. The weather is perfect for me; it's cool with sunny skies.

As we drove on Lake Shore Drive, admiring the view, Lake Michigan was breathtaking. The lake was deep blue, with a plethora of boats on the water, and seagulls circled the sky. The scenery looked like a picture painted on a canvas.

After touring Chicago briefly, Helen decided to end the sightseeing. She said she'd had enough excitement for one day. I believe the congestion, along with the traffic, and enormous size of the city, was overwhelming. We decided to seize the opportunity and go to the grocery store and purchase the food for the cookout. My family and friends were furnishing the spirits. The food preparation would take several hours. The cookout was scheduled for 1:00 p.m. and would last into the night.

The guests began arriving. I was honored to have my family and friends come out to celebrate my new beginnings in life. Everyone was excited to see me; over fifty guests had gathered, and we were having a marvelous time. There was plenty of delicious food, spirits, and wonderful company. I never realized how much I missed Chicago until I saw all my wonderful family and friends I had left behind.

I was euphoric. Everyone welcomed Helen with open arms. She is such a congenial person. She never feels like a stranger. Everyone she meets enjoys her company and becomes a friend for life. She was having a spectacular time hanging out in the back yard with my family and friends.

Night came upon us, and the guests began to leave. Helen and I were saying our goodbyes and receiving plenty of hugs and kisses.

My cousin Chip helped me with the major cleaning; it took several hours to reorganize the house and back yard. Overall, the celebration was superb and well worth the effort of traveling those fifteen hours home.

We decided to relax Sunday and enjoy our downtime. In between relaxing, I prepared us a light breakfast and a dinner that was simply scrumptious. We decided to leave for St. Louis in the morning; we were staying with my favorite cousin, Linda. We have been hanging out since we were small children. During summer vacations, my sister Natalie and I would travel to St. Louis and stay for two weeks. The temperatures were always extremely hot, and the skies were always sunny.

We would arrive in St. Louis early that morning; while we were visiting Linda, we would also be attending my dad's 1997 family reunion. The reunion was being held on my dad's birthday, which is Labor Day weekend. My Aunt Hattie was hosting the reunion that year. She has a spacious backyard with a beautiful deck. Aunt Hattie makes a delicious homemade fruit cobbler; I could not wait to taste it.

We arrived at Linda's home; we found it comfortable and cozy. The house is located in a beautiful area in the city. She has an enormous backyard with much space for her dog. Once we had settled in, we were off to Aunt Hattie's house to participate in the festivities.

When we arrived there were plenty of relatives to embrace. I spotted my dad in the crowd; he looked fantastic considering he is in his sixties but has the appearance of a man in his forties. There were plenty of birthday gifts piled on the table; I added mine to the collection.

Everyone was enjoying the festivities. Later, some of the family members went sightseeing. Without a doubt, Helen and I were enjoying our visit to St. Louis. Every precious moment that I spend with loved ones is special, and I will cherish these memories forever.

On Monday morning, we headed to Houston to visit Helen's sisters, Gwen and Teresa. This would be my first trip to Houston, and I was looking forward to meeting Helen's family. We would also visit my uncle Clinton's house.

We arrived in Houston Tuesday afternoon. Our first stop was my uncle Clinton and aunt LeNelle's house. Aunt LeNelle had prepared some delicious homemade tacos, which happens to be one of my favorite meals. I enjoy Mexican food with plenty of hot peppers, salsa, and chips.

Later, my uncle and I visited a horse ranch. I adore horses; they are one of God's most beautiful creations—so magnificent and graceful. Horses are the only creatures that have gone into battles consistently with man since wars began. When we returned, Helen and I said our goodbyes and departed.

We stayed with Helen's sister Gwen during the remainder of the trip. Besides, we were there on a mission. Helen and her sisters have a friend named Sandy who has breast cancer and refuses to get treatment. She's adamant that her church congregation can pray the cancer out of her body. She believes her strong conviction in God will heal her body of breast cancer. She was thoroughly convinced that refusing medical treatment was the right thing to do.

I believe in the power of prayer, but I also believe God gave doctors the anointing power of healing and the knowledge to assist Him in our earthly realm. I'm sure most people know of someone whose church congregation was praying the cancer or sickness out of a member's body but who nonetheless died within a year or two because the condition was never treated properly. Those same people will proclaim after the death of the member that it was God's will for that person to die. God's will was for the person to make good use of the doctors He had put in their path. And I am baffled as to why people go to the hospital for a doctor's opinion but do not follow the doctor's advice.

Later that afternoon I was introduced to Sandy. She's a beautiful, tall sister with a cocoa complexion. She could have been a runway model. We discussed her breast cancer, and I found her attitude ludicrous. She was adamant her church congregation could rid her body of cancer through prayer alone. She also informed us that she had discussed her breast cancer with her male companion and that he had stated that if she lost her breast, it would end their relationship. I told her that if he felt that way, then perhaps he wasn't worthy of her love.

I was honest about my reactions to chemotherapy and admitted I detested every moment, I also told her I felt I had made a wise decision to have the mastectomy and complete the chemotherapy. Less than thirty minutes into the conversation, Sandy began to avoid the conversation, so I ended the conversation and respected her wishes. I could only pray her decision wouldn't cost her her life!

Sandy and I spoke again Sunday morning. My persistence was futile; she did not want to discuss the breast cancer, and I had to respect her decision again. All I could do was pray Sandy would decide to have the mastectomy and chemotherapy treatments before it was too late. I let her know she could give me a call if she ever wanted to discuss the breast cancer. Sandy and I embraced, and then Helen and I said our goodbyes and departed.

As we drove down the highway, I couldn't stop thinking about Sandy's decision on the way home. I thought it would be a shame for her to lose her life at such a young age and leave behind two teenage children who depended upon her love and guidance.

Our road trip ended back home in Mobile two weeks later, and it was time for my regularly scheduled checkup with Dr. James Lawrence, the professor of rheumatology at the university. He has the appearance of a preppy college student. I was ecstatic to inform him that I hadn't experienced a lupus crisis since having chemotherapy.

Perhaps the chemotherapy did have a positive effect on my body after all and put the lupus into remission.

Dr. Lawrence has been treating me for lupus since 1994. His practice is juvenile rheumatology, but he has decided to treat adults, too. He is highly respected in this field of medicine. Dr. Lawrence has always been amazed at my positive attitude regarding lupus. I figure I shouldn't stress over an illness that has no cure. Being depressed and stressed out will not accomplish anything, nor will it change the circumstances.

Dr. Lawrence also thinks I might be in denial, because I haven't questioned God regarding having breast cancer. But who am I to question God about life?

I said to him, "Why not me? I'm no better than any other mother's or father's child on this earth. Besides, I would rather not dwell on the breast cancer. I just want to continue moving forward and managing my lupus and becoming a productive person again."

Because of my attitude, Dr. Lawrence was concerned that I may also be suffering from the medical condition bipolar disorder, more on the upside than the downside. He thought I should be depressed about the significant changes in my life: the cancer, chemotherapy, and having to close the deli. My thoughts were that that chapter in my life was over.

During my appointment, Dr. Lawrence recommended I see an oncologist for my oncology checkups for the next five years. He recommended Dr. Crane and mentioned that his nurse had already scheduled the appointment. In the meantime, I needed to have blood drawn from the lab. I prayed I wouldn't experience any drama.

Today I met Dr. Crane for the first time. She is petite and has long, curly hair. When she extended her hand to greet me, I noticed that her hands were extremely cold; they felt like ice. We discussed alternative treatments to avoid a recurrence of breast cancer due to the one lymph node that had tested positive. She had scheduled several tests: first, a chest x-ray and mammogram, and later, blood work.

I wondered if I would ever get used to having my blood drawn so frequently.

During the appointment, we also discussed the possibility of my taking a new cancer drug which was in its second year of clinical testing. I decided against the medication because of the many side effects that were associated with the drug. I'm not keen on taking medications that are still in the experimental stages.

There are always too many uncertainties involved. I felt confident that in a couple of years the laboratories would have perfected the drug; then perhaps I would consider taking the medication. And, to be honest, I'm not comfortable participating in trial studies, although I do understand the significance of participation. Because of the numerous illnesses I have, I'm apprehensive about inviting more medical chaos into my life.

My clinic appointments with Dr. Crane are scheduled every four months. During the appointments, I have a chest x-ray and a mammogram performed on the left breast. I also have lab work done on each occasion.

Usually on my first visit to a new lab, I inform the nurses and technicians of my phobia of needles. I pray for someone who is compassionate. If only I did not hear the needle when it penetrates my skin, perhaps it would be all right, but I hear a popping sound. Some people say it's psychological, but I honestly hear the needle when it breaks the skin.

However, I understand the importance of having my blood drawn; it's to detect early signs of a recurrence of breast cancer. Breast cancer can recur in various locations in the body besides the breast.

That is why early detection is so important. Early detection can help prevent the breast cancer from metastasizing. Therefore, I will willingly submit to having my blood drawn as often as required.

Eight months had passed since my mastectomy, and I no longer dressed or undressed in front of Michael. Now when I get dressed, I take my clothes either to the bathroom or one of our guestrooms. I became aware of my behavior several months ago. The reason for my behavior is that I feel abnormal only having one breast, and it appeared to be getting longer with each passing day. I believe this was occurring because the right breast was not supporting the left breast and giving it balance.

Therefore, I believed I might be suffering from low self-esteem and needed counseling to handle this situation. I was feeling incomplete and unattractive. However, I still continue to wear my loungewear because I believe in looking my best for Michael when he returns home from work. I believe sex appeal keeps a relationship interesting, so I continue maintaining the image he has grown accustomed to.

I often wished both breasts had been removed together, because then I wouldn't look and feel hideous. Sometimes I wonder if I am being punished for all those years I hated my breasts and wished they were smaller. I have learned to be careful what I wish for.

I now wondering if Michael noticed my behavior. If so, he didn't mention it. I find myself asking him frequently if he still finds me attractive, and his response is always yes. I tell myself I should accept his response and be content, but I can't!

When wearing my prosthesis, I looked and felt normal. Sometimes I even forgot I was wearing the prosthesis, because it felt natural to the touch. When I embrace people, I am sure they are unaware they are not embracing my natural breast.

I wondered how much longer I could continue this charade, pretending everything is normal. I thought, *If only I could get past these feelings of insecurity I am experiencing, I would be all right.* I know deep in my heart that having breasts does not make me a woman, but I can't stop thinking if I had my right breast I would be a whole woman again.

Because of these feelings, I scheduled an appointment with Dr. Lawrence to discuss my concerns. At that point I was sure he would recommend counseling and that this might confirm his suspicions of me being bipolar. Deep in my heart, I prayed these were normal reactions for any woman who had lost her breast because of breast cancer.

Today I had another appointment with Dr. Lawrence to discuss my return to work. I prayed that when I discussed my behavior he wouldn't recommend I see a psychiatrist. The only way a psychiatrist could understand me is if she had experienced losing a breast as well. I believe that to understand my emotions, one must walk in my shoes. People can have empathy, but they cannot fully understand my emotions.

I arrived at the clinic with a positive attitude, ready for anything Dr. Lawrence might throw my way. He surprised me with his response. He felt my emotions were normal. He believed these feelings would pass with time but suggested perhaps I should seek counseling if they didn't. He also agreed it was time to return to work, which would eliminate the idle time on my hands.

That was the best news I had received in months. As soon as I arrived home, I decided to read the classifieds and see what career opportunities were available in commission sales. Because of my apprehension regarding the long hours required to be successful, I decided to seek temporary employment until finding the right position.

I accepted a position with a temporary agency. My first assignment was with a local supermarket chain named Delfarms. The chain consists of forty grocery stores in Alabama, Mississippi, and Florida. At Delfarms Corporation, I would be assisting Ms. Brown, the customer service manager.

After my interview, I had the opportunity to meet Ms. Brown. She is in her mid sixties and has a beautiful personality. She is a well-dressed Southern belle from head to her toe.

Although it had been many years since I worked in an administrative position, I hoped to do well. I was a little apprehensive because the position involved computer skills; I have a way of destroying computers once I come in contact with them. People tell me all the time not to worry because it's difficult to break a computer, but they change their minds later. Then I get questions like, "What happened?" My response is "If I knew what caused the problem, there would not be a need for this conversation."

My first day at work was hectic. We received an abundance of calls from plenty of irate customers. In my opinion, some of the complaints could have been better handled by the managers at the stores. As the day passed, I felt confident I could do the job; however, I knew learning the position would take a couple of weeks to master.

During the course of the day, I learned Ms. Brown was well organized, which is crucial for me. I maintain a mental itinerary daily; by maintaining a schedule, my days are productive and stress free.

At lunch I met Lisa, a volunteer from the local cancer organization. She's one of the corporate executives. We shared our breast cancer experiences. She mentioned she had been dealing with some issues regarding her husband's emotional state. She expressed that he had rejected her since her mastectomies. She admitted she was having a difficult time adjusting to the situation; which would be a normal reaction for anyone. She looked as though she had been defeated; the life seemed to have been drained from her.

I can recall wondering after my mastectomy if Michael would reject me. I believe questioning whether or not your spouse will accept the drastic changes to your body is normal. Perhaps the reason some men and women have difficulties adjusting is that the change is so abrupt. Yesterday my body was normal, like every other woman's; I had two breasts. Today the only thing indicating a breast existed is a scar.

The following day, Lisa and I had lunch again. She still seemed depressed by her husband's attitude regarding the mastectomies. She was convinced he was no longer in love with her, and my heart went out to her. This was such a crucial time in her life; she needed his love and support to get through this horrific chapter in her life. I have never met the man, but if what she said was true, then perhaps she would have been better off without him. I mentioned to Lisa several times she needed to regain control of her life and to understand that her husband appeared to be having difficulty adjusting to the recent changes in their lives.

Perhaps if her husband put himself in her shoes, he would have been more considerate and compassionate. I'm sure if he were to lose an arm or a leg, he would want her to remain by his side. Sometimes I think we need to walk in each other's shoes to be more sympathetic toward each other's emotions. We never know what tomorrow may bring. We take it for granted our lives will remain the same, but life can change in a split second without any indication.

After lunch, I met an executive secretary named Grace. She's in remission with breast cancer. She appeared to be positive, energetic, and busting with life. She invited me to her office to read an article regarding her breast cancer experience. The article was featured in the local newspaper, and I found it to be enlightening. The interview had taken place on her boat as she and her mother enjoyed fishing.

Grace invited me to join her for lunch the next day, and I accepted the invitation. Meanwhile, I went back to my office to answer the telephones and keep busy so I could remain employed. I was proud of myself; I had learned the position sooner than I had anticipated, which was awesome.

When I entered the office, Ms. Brown asked if I would be interested if a permanent position became available. Of course I said yes. I couldn't say no and jeopardize my job.

The next day, it was delightful talking with Grace. Although we had just met, she was an inspiration. She spoke about keeping my sprits up and having faith in God. By doing these things, one can maintain a positive outlook on life.

Each time that Grace and I spoke, she had encouraging words.

God always knows the right time to put people in our lives, if only for a season. I mentioned to Grace that perhaps she might speak with Lisa and give her some words of encouragement. Sometimes all it takes is a special person to offer words of encouragement, and those few words can change a person's life for the better.

My heart goes out to Lisa; she does not receive the love or support from her husband which is critical in healing. Perhaps they should seek professional counseling, which would educate him on how to handle his emotions concerning Lisa losing her breasts. Then perhaps he will understand how breast cancer affects both men and women. Most men are unaware that they, too, can develop breast cancer. The breast cancer gene can be inherited from the mother and passed to the son.

I am concerned that if Lisa's situation does not improve, it will affect her ability to heal physically and mentally. Our minds play a significant part in our physical and spiritual healing. During the healing process, it's imperative to remain spiritual and positive and eliminate all negative energy.

When I returned from lunch, I was informed my position had been extended for another four months. That was terrific; it gave me the opportunity to seek full-time employment and remain employed. Although corporate work is wonderful, I've come to the realization that I enjoy working in fine furniture..

Today I had my second checkup with Dr. Crane, and all went well. My lab results were excellent, and my chest x-rays were clear. I heard all the right words I wanted to hear. I discussed the possibilities of breast reconstruction surgery. She recommended a plastic surgeon named Dr. William Thomas. He is considered one of the best reconstructive surgeons in the South. My first appointment was scheduled for December 18, 1998. And I was eagerly looking forward to my first visit.

Michael and I discussed the surgery, and he supported my decision. I found it mentally exhausting having to put my prosthesis on and remove it day after day. Besides, the law of gravity had taken complete control of my left breast; it was getting longer with each passing day. My left breast had developed into the shape of an upside-down cone; it even had a pointed tip!

Although my prosthesis was anatomically correct, it restricted me to wearing "mature" clothing because of the design of the prosthesis bras. I could no longer wear low-cut tops or spaghetti straps. It was even difficult for me to find beautiful ball gowns, because most gowns are designed with spaghetti straps or are strapless. I just wanted to feel young and attractive without having clothing restrictions in my life.

Perhaps if both breasts had been removed together, my emotions would have been more stable instead of running rampant each day. I know I should just be thankful to be alive. That's why each day when I wake up, I thank God for sparing my life. I asked Him to forgive me for wanting to make alterations to my body out of vanity.

When I returned home from work, there was a message from Custom Designs, one of the businesses where I had submitted an employment application. The company specializes in custom-designed furniture. The owner wanted to interview me for a design consultant position, and I was extremely excited. The interview was scheduled for the following week. Maybe I could start in two weeks if all went well during the interview.

Chapter Four:

Breast Reconstructive Surgery

MY FIRST APPOINTMENT WITH DR. Thomas was encouraging. He proved to be a compassionate man who was willing to listen to my concerns. His staff was unbelievably kind and went out of their way to make sure I was comfortable. We spoke in detail regarding the various operations and procedures that were available for breast reconstruction surgery.

He did, however, express his concerns regarding my history with lupus, arthritis, and the medication I was prescribed. Dr. Thomas believed a "TRAMP flap" (which involves using one of the abdominal muscles to create a breast) would not be in my best interest. Although I'm somewhat deficient on the right side because of the mastectomy, he believed he could get a tissue expander to work along with a cortral lateral reduction mammoplasty on the left breast. We discussed all the risks involved, benefits, alternatives, and imponderables that are related to breast reconstruction and breast reduction surgery.

We also discussed the risks of bleeding, infection, implant extrusion, deflation, and possible nerve damage. Dr. Thomas explained we would never get the implant perfect, and I fully understood. I was satisfied with his responses to my questions and concerns. After meeting Dr. Thomas and speaking with him, I felt I had been delivered to a child of God. A sense of peacefulness filled my soul.

The step was to take photographs of my breast for study. Then a letter was to be forwarded to the insurance company to request permission to proceed with the surgery.

Later that day I met with Mr. Mays for my interview at Custom Designs, and everything went well. I was offered the position as a design consultant, and I accepted. I was to start in two weeks. I was honest with Mr. Mays regarding my plastic surgery, which was scheduled in four weeks. This way he could make arrangements to have coverage for two days until I returned. I also explained in detail that I needed to take several days off at various times for the different procedures scheduled over the next six to nine months. However, I reassured him I would schedule the surgeries to coincide with my days off. Mr. Mays was fine with the arrangement as long as it did not interfere with business.

When Michael arrived home, we discussed the surgery again, and he supported my decision in having the procedures performed. My next consultation was scheduled for January 12, 1999, and I was ready to accept the risks involved with both procedures. I had prayed on the matter and felt confident it was the right thing to do. I desperately wanted to be a whole woman again and to stop looking and feeling hideous, as if I belonged in a circus.

During my next appointment, the sizing for the implant was determined and the tissue expander was ordered. I chose the smallest implant, which was equivalent to a 34C. I always dreamed of having smaller breasts, and now my wishes had been granted. Dr. Thomas was apprehensive about ordering the implant and expander so small; he felt I would later change my mind regarding the smaller size. I reassured him I was certain of my choice. Before I lost my breast, I wore a 38DD bra and weighed only 120lbs.

The expander and implant were to arrive the following Tuesday. The surgery was scheduled for Wednesday morning at Westside Memorial Hospital. I was scheduled for lab work on Tuesday to ensure it was safe to perform the operation. I felt positive everything would be all right.

On the morning of the surgery, I asked to speak with my surgical team. I wanted to make sure everyone was having a terrific day and we were all on one accord. After all, I was putting my life into the hands of strangers again, and I needed some reassurances. The surgery was considered an outpatient procedure, so I would be discharged when Dr. Thomas determined I was not experiencing any life-threatening complications.

I was in recovery for several hours and then released. On the way home, we stopped and had the pain medication prescription filled. I did not know if I would experience side effects; therefore, I had requested a few days off from work to allow myself time to recover. When we arrived home I undressed and prepared for bed. I had no idea how drastically my life was about to change.

Several hours later, I was consumed with the most awful pain imaginable. The saline solution was beginning to fill out the expander. My chest felt as if a ton of bricks had fallen upon it and there was no relief in sight.

When the expander began to expand, the pressure became unbearable. All I could do was cry and ask God to forgive me for making alterations to my body out of vanity.

The pain medication provided no relief. I sat on the end of the daybed in our guestroom. I cried as I held myself and rocked. No one had prepared me for the excruciating pain I was experiencing. I prayed to God and asked Him to forgive me, and I promised God that if I survived this crisis, I would never again make any alterations to my body except to save my life. I believed I had committed the worst sin imaginable. Michael felt defenseless; there wasn't anything he could do to alleviate the pain. At one time, I was in such excruciating pain he wanted to take me back to the hospital to have the expander removed. I told him no; I felt the pain eventually would subside.

Meanwhile I had already taken four pain pills trying to gain relief. And after several hours, the pain began to dissipate. The medication was beginning to provide relief. I guess my body was in shock from the foreign device that had invaded my chest, and the anesthesia had begun to wear off. My next appointment was scheduled for January 29, 1999. If all went well, I would have the sutures removed from the breast reduction. I also planned on informing Dr. Thomas of the excruciating pain I had experienced.

When Saturday arrived, all I could do was lie in bed. The pain continued throughout the weekend. I had many thoughts of regret regarding the surgery. I wondered if I had made the correct decision, but it was too late; the harm was already done. And I would just have to deal with the pain. Yet again, I felt I was being punished for the numerous times I wished I had smaller breasts. I was supposed to accept my breasts and appreciate what God had given me.

Two weeks passed, and it was time for my clinic appointment. My incision was healing beautifully, and the sutures were removed. I shared my horrific pain experience with Dr. Thomas. He assured me I should not experience any more severe pain. He did, however, explain I would experience discomfort while going through the expansion process. After hearing that information, we both decided another pain prescription would be in order. I wanted to be prepared for my next injection, which was scheduled in three weeks.

Meanwhile, my body had become acquainted with the breast expander that was now an "extended guest." I continued to pray and ask God for His forgiveness. There were still several surgeries and procedures required. They involved the expander transfer, insertion of the implant, and the left breast reduction procedure to balance my chest. During my next appointment, it would be a bit difficult to inflate the expander. The saline solution would be injected into the tissue expander while I was conscious.

I was also horrified to learn each injection would be administered through a button inserted underneath my skin next to the expander during the surgery. I must have been out of my mind to agree to have this procedure performed, but I guess that's what vanity does. Again I learned to be careful of what I wished for. I never once considered how the expander would increase in size. At that moment I realized I had not done enough research regarding the breast implant procedure.

I'm sure Dr. Thomas explained what the procedure involved, but apparently I did not comprehend the information that was given.

For my next appointment, I arrived thirty minutes prior to my appointment. I had the opportunity to spend time in the waiting area.

There were quite a few patients waiting to be seen by different plastic surgeons.

As I sat there, waiting patiently for my name to be called, I was intrigued by the number of people present. I tried to determine what type of surgery each person had had or would be having. With some of the patients, it was quite obvious.

While observing the area, I noticed a young man about fifteen years old who was trying desperately to isolate himself from everyone. After taking only a quick glance, one would wonder why he was there. Then I noticed the left side of his skull was caved in. I was curious as to what caused this devastation. I was compelled to speak to him. He was shy but was intelligent and polite. I'm sure he was praying for a miracle from God.

Once the young man was called, I noticed another gentleman sitting; he had some sort of green growth in the form of a ball located between his eyes and nose. I had never seen anything like it. After observing several more patients, it was obvious that the majority of these people were disfigured and required plastic surgery.

After making my observation of the waiting area, I was called and taken to the examining room. There was a small cart set up with surgical tools for the procedure. The first injection took about thirty minutes to perform. Dr. Thomas and I talked the entire time to distract my mind from the procedure. I never expected to see the needle, but it was unavoidable. I guess we live and learn from our mistakes, and this was a lesson I would never forget.

On my way home, the saline solution began to fill the expander out and caused a tremendous amount of pain. I literally drove home resting on the steering wheel. I prayed I would not get pulled over by the police. How was I going to explain the situation; things weren't clear to me! The drive home felt like an eternity. I asked myself if I could endure another injection. I knew I would be in constant prayer for the next six months. When I arrived home, all I could do was lie across the bed and thank God I'd had the pain prescription filled. I took several pills and tossed and turned for several hours before the medication took effect.

Once again I began to have second thoughts regarding the reconstructive surgery and the breast implant. After each injection, the pressure increased as a result of the additional saline solution. I prayed for the strength to continue. I was scheduled to see Dr. Thomas once a week, and honestly, I was reluctant.

I was reluctant regarding sharing my painful experiences with Michael. I did not want to alarm him; he would have taken off work to ensure my safe return home.

Several months had passed since I began the reconstruction surgery. On March 23, 1999, two days before my forty-first birthday, I had a clinic appointment with my oncologist. I had concerns regarding the density in my incision I had dicovered around the reconstructed area. There appeared to be a mass in the area. My first thoughts were, *If I am experiencing a recurrence of breast cancer, this is the worst timing imaginable.* I still needed several treatments to complete the reconstructive breast surgery and had never imagined the possibility of having to discontinue the procedure, but I would do what was in the best interest of my health.

I shared my concerns regarding the recurrence with Dr. Crane. She agreed I should have an ultrasound performed on the right side to determine if I was experiencing a recurrence. I decided to wait for the x-ray results, which would only take an hour. Meanwhile, I was going out of my mind, pacing the hallways. When the radiology nurse called my name, I could barely move my feet. I was praying for the courage to be strong.

The radiologist said that the ultrasound demonstrated normal breast tissue and that there was no evidence of a recurrence or any other abnormality. I would be able to enjoy the rest of the day and share my wonderful news with Michael. I thought that by the time I finished with the surgeries and procedures I would have aged twenty years. My courage and faith were being tested, and I prayed to be worthy enough to come out a winner.

Tonight we will celebrate my forty-first birthday with friends over dinner. Michael knows I adore gold bracelets, so he left a stunning bracelet on my pillow. At dinner I announced that there were no signs of a recurrence of breast cancer. This indeed was an occasion for a celebration.

A week later I was back at the clinic for another injection. There were several people in the waiting area. I found myself inquisitive again as to why everyone was there. There was a toddler with two black eyes due to a surgical procedure. I was amazed at all the patients waiting to be seen. The nurse finally called my name and led me to the examining room. The surgical instruments required for the procedure were laid out and ready to go. Forty-five ccs of saline were added to the expander. Once again, Dr. Thomas spoke with me regarding the risks, benefits, and alternatives. My next appointment was scheduled for two weeks later, and then we would schedule the next surgical procedure, which would remove the expander and replace it with the breast implant.

Again, I was grateful I had taken the pain medication prior to leaving home. When I returned home, I took another pain pill and prepared for bed. Having the procedures performed on my off days allows my body the opportunity to adjust to the drastic transformation, which takes twenty-four hours to complete.

Mr. Mays surprised us today and brought his daughter to work. She was a beautiful three year old. She had short, curly hair and was full of energy. After a few minutes of observation, I noticed an abnormal growth on her face. She looked as if she had sustained several serious burns. I later learned she was born with red marks on her face and back that had developed into abnormal growths. Some of the growths were as large as a quarter and were reddish and green in color. All I could do was imagine this child growing up with these abnormal growths covering her body and being teased by the other children. On my next appointment with Dr. Thomas, I planned to ask him if he was aware of this particular condition.

On April 13 I had my preoperative consultation with Dr. Thomas. We discussed the risks associated with the procedures, which involved the actual implant exchange, the inferior reposition of the nipple, and the left reduction mammoplasty. I was anxious and ready to get the surgery behind me; it was time for me to move forward in my life. And I was sure Michael would be ecstatic when the drama was behind us. Although he never once complained, I know he was affected emotionally by the situation.

When the consultation ended, Dr. Thomas and I discussed Mr. Mays's daughter's condition. He felt that if he could examine her, he possibly could assist her. He suggested I try to get a picture, if possible. I hoped Mr. Mays would not be offended that I had spoken with Dr. Thomas regarding his daughter's condition. I was certain that although she was only three, she felt different from the other children. In my opinion, it would be an injustice not to reveal the beauty this child possessed.

Deep in my heart, I felt it was the proper thing to do.

After returning to work, I mentioned to Mr. Mays that I had spoken with Dr. Thomas regarding his daughter's condition, that I had described her condition to the best of my ability, and that Dr. Thomas thought he could better assess her condition if he had a photo. I assured Mr. Mays Dr. Thomas was confident he could assist her through plastic surgery. Mr. Mays agreed to give me a picture. He was appreciative of my concern for his daughter's well-being.

On the morning of surgery, I was experiencing anxiety attacks. The procedure was considered outpatient surgery; I planed to be discharged in several hours if there were no complications. The insurance companies approved the outpatient surgery because it decreases the medical cost significantly. In my opinion, I believe quality medical care should be the main objective in medical treatments, but I am a realist and understand it's all about the bottom-line profits.

My thoughts were that I should remain in the hospital at least overnight for observation. I was considering having the expander removed; the implant inserted into my chest and breast reduction performed on the left breast. I prayed everything would go well. I requested to speak with the surgical team before surgery. I wanted to make certain everyone involved was having a super day. I asked my routine questions regarding what type of morning everyone was experiencing.

I discussed with Dr. Thomas the possibility of eliminating the Jackson-Pratt drainage bottles. I explained I was unable to deal with the excruciating pain associated with the removal of the drainage bottles. We reached an agreement: if I retained fluids, he would have to insert the drainage bottles to reduce the chances of an infection.

I prayed he was a man of his word and would keep his promise. I strongly believed I would only retain a minimum amount of fluid, thereby eliminating the need for the drainage bottles.

After regaining consciousness, the first thing I asked Michael was whether there were any drainage bottles on my sides, and he replied by saying no. I regained consciousness and repeated the same question. He reassured me there were no drainage bottles, and apparently I lost consciousness again. On my third awakening, I stayed conscious. I finally took both hands and ran them down my sides, making sure there were no drainage bottles. When I realized there were no bottles, I thanked God for Dr. Thomas keeping his promise.

I remained in recovery for two hours, and then a nurse assisted me in getting dressed. I tried to explain I had not fully recovered. She just looked at me and continued with her assistance. Once I was fully dressed, she helped me into the wheelchair and asked Michael where he was parked. She stated she would meet him outside. She immediately wheeled me to the entrance, and when Michael drove up, he assisted me into the vehicle.

Apparently I had dozed off several times during the drive home, because it seems as if I kept losing time.

I must admit it was fantastic to be going home; I knew all my needs would be met. And once again my chest felt as if a ton of bricks had fallen on it. On the way home, Michael stopped at the drug store to purchase the pain medication. When we arrived home, I immediately took two pills, undressed, and went to bed. I could barely keep my eyes open because of the anesthesia.

Michael woke me later for supper and checked to make sure I did not have a fever or was experiencing any complications. I informed him I was fine but was experiencing some pressure and discomfort in my chest. I remember thinking how blessed I was having a devoted husband. We talked for a while, and I fell asleep.

Chapter Five:

A New Beginning

SEVERAL WEEKS PASSED, AND IT came time for my symmetry evaluation. My symmetry was much improved. The sutures on my right breast and the staples from the reduction were removed.

The following Tuesday I would return to have the areola sutures removed from the nipple area. Because my natural breasts were so large, the nipple had to be removed, altered in size, and then repositioned back onto the breast. I discovered the snipping of my nipple had made it sensitive to touch. I found it to be stimulating!

When I returned to work the following day, I had excellent news for Mr. Mays. I informed him Dr. Thomas had reviewed the pictures and was aware of the condition. He recommended Mr. Mays and his wife bring their daughter in for evaluation. Dr. Thomas positively believed he could remove the abnormal growths from her face and her back. Mr.

Mays immediately called his wife, and they made the appointment for the following Monday.

Mr. and Mrs. Mays met with Dr. Thomas. They decided to have the surgery performed on Wednesday. Dr. Thomas assured them that when he surgically removed the growth it would not return and that their daughter could lead a normal, healthy life and do all the things little girls do, such as use makeup, go to parties and dances, and just hang out with friends.

I was ecstatic at the wonderful news and proud to be a part of this young girl's life. I believe we all play an intricate role in each other's lives because we are all connected through Jesus Christ, our Lord. God is always on time; He knows just who to put in our lives at the appropriate time. Who would have thought my plastic surgery would be central to Mr. Mays's daughter? Sometimes all it takes is one season to bring about a spectacular change in someone's life, and when that event occurs, cherish the moment.

After the major reconstruction of the surgery was completed, I decided to take the opportunity to enroll in an interior decorating course. A diploma could prove to be beneficial for my career. There is a high demand for decorators on the Gulf Coast. There are thousands of condominiums owned by northerners, whom we refer to as snowbirds. The snowbirds spend an enormous amount of time and money on the Gulf Coast during the fall and winter months. During the spring and summer, they rent out their condominiums. The beautifully decorated condos bring in enormous profits for the investors and excellent commissions for the realtors.

The weekend for the reunion came, and Michael and I arrived in Houston late Friday afternoon, along with many other relatives, for our 1999 family reunion. We were staying at the Ramada Inn Resort, a beautiful, centrally-located hotel with all the amenities. My mother and my sister Natalie were flying in from Chicago and St. Louis. I was looking forward to seeing my two favorite cousins, Linda and Tyrone.

Aunt LeNelle and Uncle Clinton had planned plenty of activities for the weekend. I impatiently waited for the festivities to get started, hoping this year I could participate in all the events. I prayed for a low heat index, which would permit me to stay outdoors during the picnic.

Upon our arrival, we discovered my cousin's wife, Joyce, had breast cancer and was undergoing chemotherapy. The cancer had metastasized throughout her entire body. She was not expected to live the year out. She was only thirty-eight years old, with a teenage son graduating from high school. He had received a four-year scholarship, and chances were Joyce would not see him graduate.

I admired Joyce's courage; she handled her situation superbly. She was speaking positively despite her prognosis. She still had hopes of a miracle. Joyce was glowing, full of life. Her makeup was beautiful, and her outfit was impeccable. Anyone could tell she was at peace with God and herself. She was my heroine and role model. My heart goes out to her loved ones, and I will keep her son in my prayers.

Saturday's picnic was splendid! The heat index was perfect; I guess the praying helped. We had an excellent turnout. There was plenty of delicious food along with wonderful socializing; we enjoyed ourselves. There were relatives as young as three months and as old as ninety-eight years of age. It's amazing how active the seniors still are, and their memories are keen. Aunt Mandy is in her nineties and blind, but she can still distinguish all her nieces' and nephews' voices. I wish my memory were as keen; it's difficult for me to remember someone's name on the first or second encounter.

After the picnic, we returned to our room to relax. I was anxious to see the events planned for the evening. Tonight would be my first opportunity to wear a spaghetti-strap gown since my mastectomy.

The gown is black satin with a split just above the knee, along with matching accessories.

Michael and I had dozed off to sleep. Had it not been for my nephews Eugene and Anthony knocking on the door, we might have slept through the banquet. We hurried to get dressed. I felt incredibly attractive and looked magnificent. I was feeling glamorous; my youth had been restored.

When we arrived, Aunt LeNelle was handing out awards for various categories, such as the most reunions attended, the oldest family member, and graduation awards. The hotel staff had done an outstanding job decorating the banquet hall. There was plenty of delicious food; some was Cajun, which was quite spicy. There was a live band that performed until the banquet ended.

We took plenty of photographs and exchanged telephone numbers with those who were participating for the first time. It's astonishing to celebrate four generations of families during one occasion. After the banquet ended, we decided to hang out at a bar. We were having a terrific time just talking and passing the time away. We knew the morning would be the last time some of us would see each other until the next reunion in 2001. Every minute was a precious moment we wanted to treasure.

On Sunday morning, we all gathered for the breakfast buffet. There were plenty of delicious goodies. We talked, laughed, and had a marvelous time. As time went by, we began to check out of the hotel and head for our destinations. Some people had driven and some had flown; we even had some arrive by train and bus. Michael and I were fortunate, as Mobile was only an eight-hour drive away.

On August 10, 1999, I was at the clinic, having nipple reconstructive surgery performed on my right breast. The procedure was performed under local anesthesia. I watched as Dr. Thomas began the procedure.

Wow! I was mesmerized while watching Dr. Thomas as he inserted the needle into my right breast and withdrew a small portion of skin. He then tied the sutures around the skin until it developed into the form of a rosebud. Watching the nipple form was remarkable; the procedure took an hour to complete.

After the nipple procedure, I was scheduled for my regularly oncology checkup. I spoke with Dr. Crane again concerning my suspicions regarding a recurrence. My instincts were becoming extremely strong, and usually they are correct. I was not sure what to do. I thought about seeking another medical opinion but dreaded getting acquainted with a new doctor and staff. It can be mentally as well as physically exhausting. On my way home, I prayed for God to rid my body of the cancer.

A few days later, I returned to the clinic to retrieve my medical records. I was anxious to study the report regarding my medical condition. Perhaps there was something in the pathology report Dr. Crane overlooked. The mass appeared to be increasing in size. I could feel it in the incision, and

I was horrified by its presence. I continued to pray the entire weekend, asking God to rid my body of the dreadful cancer disease.

On Sunday evening, I finally had the opportunity to read my medical report from my previous appointment. When I read the report, something just did not seem right with the report; the report reads as follows:

PATIENT: BRENDA E. ROCKER

Patient is an African-American female, 41 years old asymptomatic female. She is status post right mastectomy for infiltrating ductal carcinoma in the past. The patient has had interval breast reduction surgery. There are scattered fibro-glandular densities in the left breast that could obscure a lesion on the mammography. There are no masses, micro-calcifications, architectural distortion, skin or nipple changes, or auxiliary adenopathy.

IMPRESSION Birads Category negative mammogram left breast. No evidence of malignancy. Recommend repeat mammogram in one year.

END OF REPORT

When I finished reading the medical report, I had concerns regarding the scattered fibro-glandular densities in the left breast. Deep in my heart, I knew I was experiencing a recurrence of breast cancer. I was trying not to become alarmed, but how could I not be concerned when I knew my suspicions were correct? This situation was becoming more nerve wracking each day.

My next appointment with Dr. Thomas was made to complete the nipple procedure. When I arrived, I wanted to have a positive outlook, but my spirits were down. I prayed the nipple tattooing under local anesthetic would take only an hour. Dr. Thomas chose the color pigments required for my complexion. He combined them to achieve the correct tone for my nipple. The colors chosen were fascinating as well as intriguing, because they were red, yellow, brown, and blue. Once the pigments were mixed properly, they matched my complexion perfectly. The procedure only took an hour; there was little discomfort involved. We were getting closer to completing the breast reconstruction, which would make me a whole woman again.

I was relieved I had requested the day off, because my mind was filled with despair. I couldn't stop thinking about the medical report.

I found the report bewildering. Could the fibrous tissue be obscuring the lesion, or was my imagination working overtime?

When I arrived home, I took a shower and tried to relax. I wanted this day to end as quickly as possible. I was hoping that I was experiencing a terrible nightmare and that when I awakened this day would never have happened. I could only hope the new year would bring about a change in my health.

I retrieved my medical records from November 16, 1999. I felt anxious about the nodule (small mass) I was positive was there. When I read the report, it seemed to contradict what my oncologist stated.

DEPARTMENT OF RADIOLOGY
PATIENT: Brenda E. Rocker November 16, 1999
ULTRASOUND STUDY OF LEFT BREAST: 11/16 /99

CLINICAL DATA: The patient is referred by Oncologist having palpated a tiny nodule just beneath the scar at the medial aspect of the breast. This is the site of previous breast reduction. The small nodule is palpable at the medial end of the scar.

On ultrasound examination this small lesion is hypoechoic and measures 4.4 mm at its greatest diameter. This may well be a suture granuloma or inclusion cyst. It has a benign appearance.

More medial and above the scar is an ill-defined palpable area that has the feeling of fibrosis or scarring subcutaneously. On examination this lesion is hypoechoic or complex and measures 13.6 mm in greatest diameter. I feel the lesion has benign characteristics on ultrasound and should be observed closely by clinical examination.

There are no purely solid lesions identified.

Mammogram images and reports are kept on fi le in patient's permanent folder.

NOTE: The results of this mammogram were communicated to the patient, verbally and written, before she left the Breast Center.

END OF REPORT

When New Year's Day 2000 arrived, my fears of a recurrence of breast cancer had not changed. I assumed that by now my doctors and others thought I was a hypochondriac. And because of the uncertainties, I was stressed out and experiencing more frequent anxiety attacks followed by lupus episodes. So I decided to request time off from work; I was unable to concentrate.

I thanked God that I had Michael's support.

Later that day, I was consumed with my own "pity party" until I received a telephone call from Aunt LeNelle. She shared with me that Joyce had succumbed to breast cancer; she had died at home in the presence of her loved ones. Joyce was only thirty-nine years old, and I believe if she had been diagnosed sooner she might still be alive today. She will be greatly missed by everyone. I'm sure God will be watching over her son and will see him through his journey in life.

My annual oncology and gynecology examinations were performed, and they appeared to be normal. Dr. Crane and I spoke again concerning the mass, and we discussed the possibilities of me taking the current cancer blocker that was available. Once again, I decided against the drug because of the numerous side effects.

I tried hard to remain positive but could not eliminate the daily thoughts of a recurrence of breast cancer, and depression had settled in. I believe Dr. Crane dismissed my concerns because I questioned her judgment. I concluded that perhaps I needed a reality check and should get a second opinion to relieve my mind. Each time I had an appointment with my oncologist, I wondered if that day would be the day I would be diagnosed with a recurrence.

After receiving my interior decorator diploma today. I decided, since I was still on leave from Custom Designs, this was the opportunity to apply for a decorating position. I chosen to wear a two-piece navy suit along with matching handbag and shoes. After all, there is only one time to make a good first impression

I was nervous as I drove to Branson's and was praying I would make a good first impression. When I entered the store, I was spellbound. Never before had I seen such exquisite furniture. I remember thinking how magnificent everything appeared; It was just like a picture on the front cover of a magazine.

I filled out an application and spoke briefly with the manager and left my resumé. He stated they did indeed need a decorator. He also said that if they were interested, he would give me a call. I thanked him for his time and said I looked forward to hearing from him. As I walked to my car, I said a prayer and asked God to bless me with the decorating position.

When I arrived home, I immediately checked my messages. To my surprise, there was a message from the manager at Branson's. He asked me to give him a call to schedule an interview. I promptly returned the call. He asked if the interview could be scheduled for the following day; my first impression had been a good one.

I prepared my clothes for the next day's interview. I wanted everything to be perfect. I planned to arrive fifteen to twenty minutes prior to the interview, making sure I was well prepared. I planned to take my diploma just in case the manager needed verification. The interview was scheduled for 10:00 a.m., which was fantastic, because I prefer mornings. The anticipation of the next day's interview consumed my every thought.

During the interview, the manager offered me the decorator position. I was to start in two weeks. I was elated that I had successfully landed my first interior decorating position.

Chapter Six:

The Accident

NUMEROUS CHANGES OCCURRED IN MY life during the previous year. I had completed my breast reconstructive surgery and resigned from Branson's. Before resigning, I learned of the finest furniture and accessories in decorating. I had taken a position at Harlem's Fine Furniture, where I was earning a fantastic salary with excellent benefits. I had also been offered a decorator's position with Don Taylor's Fine Furniture. The store had only been in existence for six months and was owned by a local family. I was offered an excellent salary and commission. The hours were wonderful, and I must admit I adored the idea of having the opportunity to decorate and purchase furniture for a 20,000-square-foot showroom.

Now that my career was back on track, we decided to purchase a home; we had outgrown our townhouse. I had discovered a charming house in our neighborhood, only a couple of blocks from where we were living. I'd looked at the house several times from the outside and was sure the interior was as adorable and charming as the exterior. I thought the house would make a terrific investment.

It was 1,700 square feet, sat on a half-acre of land, and had a beautiful back yard, a workshop, and a storage building. There were plenty of trees located on the property, and there was also a beautiful patio outlined with plush hedges. The house was empty and available for occupancy.

Although Michael and I had initially discussed building a 2,200-square-foot home, I was mysteriously drawn to this particular house.

A voice inside of my head was telling me this was the house for us. When Michael arrived home, I asked if we could take a look at the house. The location was perfect, but he believed the house was inadequate because of its size. He did like the workshop, because he enjoys working with wood.

I could imagine the shop lined with power tools and him spending a significant amount of time out there, but he still wanted the option of viewing other homes or building a house. I agreed, so he gave Barbara, our realtor, a call. Amazingly, she had several homes on the market. We agreed to meet the following day.

I am sure Barbara was astonished to learn we were seriously considering purchasing a home. Michael and I had started house hunting eight years before, but we never had any luck. Everything had to be perfect; the trees and shrubbery had to be located in a particular area of the lawn or the land had to be picture perfect. I had finally given up and refused to continue house hunting with him.

Unfortunately, Michael and I couldn't reach an agreement on any of the homes we were shown. The houses were 2,000 square feet or more, but for various reasons, they did not appeal to me. Barbara decided to locate more listings for the following day.

On our way home, Michael and I decided to take another look at the house. When he parked the car, I knew it was useless; he had not changed his mind. He was adamant regarding my obsession with furniture and feared we would outgrow the house in a few years. I promised not to fill the house with wall-to-wall furniture and allow walking space in each room. He still insisted the house was insufficient but agreed to take another look. That night, before going to bed, I prayed we would be blessed with the house. I prayed nothing else would appeal to us.

The following morning, Barbara faxed several listings to Michael, who called me and said there were several houses he thought would be sufficient. One was located near my job, so we decided to meet Barbara during lunch. The first house we viewed was a beautiful 2,200-square-foot house on an acre of land that had an enormous back yard with a huge swimming pool. I was uneasy about the pool; I could imagine someone drowning. The patio was a concern as well; it sat about ten feet higher than the other property on the same lot. The master bedroom patio looked down onto the swimming pool.

I knew finding a home with Michael was going to be a long, drawn-out process, and I wasn't looking forward to the challenges that lay ahead.

Later that evening we met with Barbara to view other listings that Michael had requested. Once we finished viewing those houses, we drove to the house I preferred. Again, it was pointless; he wasn't interested. Michael disliked the inside of the house; it was too small, and he also disliked the design of the great room. I wished he would change his mind once he viewed the workshop, but it was futile, and his answer remained no.

We continued to look, but it was pointless; my mind was set only on one house, and ironically, Michael was against the purchase.

Some of the other houses we viewed needed remodeling and would take several months of work before we could move in. To build a house would take four to six months. Before driving home, I suggested we take another look at the house, hoping Michael would have a change of heart. I hinted it would make an excellent anniversary gift and a wonderful birthday present. He agreed to give Barbara a call in the morning for another look. I felt confident that if I could get him to take another look at the property, I could persuade him to purchase the house.

Only time would tell!

It worked! In the morning, we took another look at the house and decided to make an offer. All day I tried to remain focused, but it was impossible. I was counting down the hours, waiting for Michael to call to inform me if the sellers accepted the offer. Michael finally called, but with disappointing news: the sellers needed to think about the offer. I prayed the sellers would accept the offer. The house had been on the market for nine months, and the owners had relocated to Birmingham. Finally, I received the wonderful news I had been waiting to hear: the sellers had agreed to accept the offer.

This was the first week of March 2001, and we anticipated our closing by the end of the month. I knew there was plenty of packing ahead, but I was anticipating the challenges. I planned to pack in the evenings and on my days off.

The next day, after work, I began packing and preparing for the move. I decided to hire a moving company to assist with the move. I had a list of moving companies to call for rates. Michael said he would speak with several of his friends and see if they could assist in the move, so we couldn't go wrong either way. I planned for the transition to be smooth and organized.

However, when I called several moving companies, I was appalled at the rates. Therefore, I decided against hiring a company. Michael's friends Jef and Jenkins agreed to assist with the move. Meanwhile, I continued packing. I wanted everything to be ready once we closed on the house.

However, I had never realized the abundance of glasses I had accumulated over the past twenty-one years. There must have been over three hundred glasses, not including the china, crystal, and everyday dishes we used. I started collecting glasses in 1983, when I lived in Germany, and the collection had continued to multiply over the years. I just enjoyed collecting beautiful stemware, especially fine crystal. When I began to pack, I soon realized I needed additional boxes to accommodate all the glasses.

We closed on the house and began moving on March 28, anticipating a smooth transition. Michael, Jef, and Jenkins were well organized.

They listened to my suggestions on which items to pack and which items needed to be handled with exceptional care. I acquired an elegant crystal cocktail table I had custom-designed when living in Germany. The table has sentimental value and is a one-of-a-kind piece. The top is crystal and is outlined with two beveled lines that intersect all four corners; a brass bar holds together the four crystal legs. The bar alone weighs thirty pounds. Because of the weight of the top, it requires three to four people to handle.

Once the guys left the townhouse, I continued packing the glasses. I was unaware Michael had taken the ladder, leaving me nothing to stand on to reach the cabinet above the refrigerator. I decided to climb on top of the kitchen counter to reach the cabinet.

Once the counter was full, I planned to climb down and pack the glasses into the boxes. Unfortunately, it did not turn out that way. While standing on the countertop reaching above the refrigerator, I slipped and fell into the corner of the freezer door. I realized my breast reduction had been injured, and I was experiencing excruciating pain and couldn't move. I remained on top of the refrigerator for twenty minutes before I could climb down. The pain was agonizing!

When I finally climbed down off the counter, I was able to lie on the kitchen floor, still in an immense amount of pain. The telephones had been disconnected, and I was without my cell phone, which made it impossible to contact Michael to inform him of my distress. A half an hour passed before I was able to make it to the car. I was blessed we had moved only a few blocks away. I entered the house doubled over in pain. Michael asked what had happened. I explained the situation, and he immediately examined my incision and determined all was fine. I decided to finish unpacking the following day, which was Sunday.

I lay down for the remainder of the day and later took a shower and prepared for bed. During the night, I was restless because of the awful pain I was experiencing. I knew I had injured myself worse than I imagined. I prayed the pain would soon subside. The pain reminded me of the breast reconstruction surgery. Luckily I had pain medication left over from surgery, so I decided to take some.

Shortly after taking two pills, I finally fell asleep, only to waken a short time later from the terrible pain. All I could do was cry as I rocked myself. The pain was so intense it did not allow me to sleep through the night.

On Sunday morning, as we prepared for church, I was still experiencing pain. I decided to continue unpacking and arranging the furniture when we returned from church. I knew it was going to be an all-day task. The most tedious chore would be unpacking over four hundred miniature figurines I had collected over the past twenty-one years. Each time I handle the figurines, I discover something new and exciting. The craftsmanship is exceptional. Each piece is fascinating; the collection consists of Precious Moments figures, miniature candy jars, and two one-inch red Chevrolet Corvettes.

By nightfall I had the entire house arranged, and everything was in its proper place; I was satisfied: it looked just as I had imagined. The only room without furniture was the living room. We had gained two additional rooms. We were able to furnish our dinning room, because I had been given an antique formal dining room set from my cousin Nanette who inherited it. The set fit perfectly in the dining room. The table belonged to her grandmother, then her mother. I could not avoid purchasing living room furniture because we had acquired a den.

Today is April 5, 2001 I had my four-and-a-half year checkup with Dr. Crane. During the examination I explained the injury I had sustained to my breast reduction. Dr. Crane examined my breast and determined the incision had been bruised but not torn. She stated there were no signs of recurrence of breast cancer.

This was the happiest day in my life. I could finally relax; after all these years wondering if I would survive the next five years.

And now I was only six months away from being cancer free, a cancer survivor's dream. If one survives five years, chances are he or she has beaten breast cancer, which is a survivor's ultimate goal.

That was the best news I had received in several years.

The anticipation of sharing my magnificent and exciting news with Michael and my family and friends was exhilarating. By then the medical staff at the cancer center was accustomed to me picking up my medical records. Now that I was cancer free, perhaps I could finally put my mind at ease and enjoy the rest of my life.

Several days had passed since my appointment. I notified the records department I would be picking up my latest records. I looked forward to reading these particular medical reports, as I was finally cancer free. No words could express the joy I was experiencing.

After reviewing my medical documents, I was relieved as I read each page.

The next several pages are copies of the actual medical reports.

CLINIC NOTE APRIL 5, 2001
ROCKER, BRENDA DOB: 3/25/58
CHART# 0000000000
PATIENT PROFILE: The patient is a 42-year-old African-

American woman followed for stage II carcinoma of the breast whose history is summarized on my notes of August 12, 1997. The patient presents for disease re-assessment.

SUBJECTIVE: Ms. Rocker has been well and has no complaints suggestive of recurrence of breast cancer. She has no symptoms suggestive toxicity from prior cancer-directed therapy. She has had an injury to the left breast (a fall), and has soreness in the area of the incision of the prior reduction surgery. She has no neurological, respiratory, gastrointestinal, cardiac, or bony complaints.

CHRONIC MEDICATIONS:

1. Lupus medication 400 milligrams P.O. q day.

2. Antidepressant 50 milligrams P.O. q hs.

3. Antidepressant prn.

4. Iron 325 milligrams P.O. bid.

OBJECTIVE: Weight 143.5 pounds, temperature 96.3, and blood pressure 120/80, and pulse 90, SWOG performance status of 0. In general the patient is a medium-build, African-American woman in no apparent distress. HEENT examination is unremarkable, no oral lesions. Neck is supple without supraclavicular or cervical adenopathy. There is no tenderness over the bony spine. Lungs are clear bilaterally. Heart is regular without murmur.

The right chest wall is status post reconstruction and without obvious evidence for local recurrence. The left breast was status post surgical reduction. There is no axillary adenopathy. The medial aspect of the incision of the left breast is with a bruise. There is no mass.

The liver is percussed to be approximately 6 centimeters in the mid-clavicular line today. No inguinal or epitrochlear adenopathy. No lower extremity edema.

LABORATORY DATA: CBC is remarkable for hemoglobin of 97.7 Chemistry panel is negative.

ASSESSMENT:

1. T2 (two primaries: 1.2 centimeters and 1.5 centimeters) N1 (1/18nodes positive) M0 infiltration ductal carcinoma in this premenopausal woman, status post modified radical mastectomy on February 10, 1997. ER was 3+ and PgR 3+ on both primaries visa assay on paraffin blocks. The patient was treated with four cycles of chemotherapy given by Dr. Mann. The patient transferred her care to our center August of 1997. Adjuvant Tamoxifen has been subsequently been discussed with the patient and a trial was attempted. Due to poor tolerance the patient opted to discontinue.

2. Iron deficiency anemia, diagnosed in February of 1998.

3. Undifferentiated connective tissue disease.

4. Status post herpes zosters on back left leg in June of 1997.

5. Reported reactions to codeine with various reported reactions.

6. Status post left breast reduction and right chest reconstruction in 1999.

PLAN:

1. No specific therapy is recommended for the trauma to the left breast from the fall. I advised the patient this should resolve.

2. The patient is to continue with annual mammography.

3. Serum iron, total iron binding capacity, and ferritin were added on the patient's laboratory to ensure that this is still consistent with iron deficiency.

Division of Hematology/Oncology

END OF REPORT

HSF DEPARTMENT OF RADIOLOGY
NAME: Rocker, Brenda Date of Birth: 03/25 /1958
X-ray # Date: 04/5 /2001
ROENTGENOLOGICAL FINDING
PA AND LATERAL VIEWS OF THE CHEST: 4/5/2001

CLINICAL HISTORY: Breast cancer.

Comparison is made with the previous study from 9/12/2000.

There has been no change in the appearance of the heart, lungs or mediastinum. Again seen is partial mastectomy on the right side.

There is no evidence of metastasis disease.

END OF REPORT

Chapter Seven:

Recurrence of Breast Cancer

SEVERAL MONTHS HAD PASSED SINCE the injury occurred to my breast, and I was experiencing some discomfort. I believed there was a reason to be concerned, and I used a mirror to observe the injury myself. I was astounded to discover a hairline tear. The tear was about a quarter inch long and was so thin it could be overlooked with only a quick glance. I immediately called Dr. Thomas, my plastic surgeon, and expressed my concerns. He recommended I come the following morning.

The next morning, I met with Dr. Thomas. He asked when the injury had occurred. I replied, "The last week in March." It was then the end of July. By the expression upon his face, I could sense something was seriously wrong. He spoke those dreaded words I had feared hearing. He suspected I was experiencing a recurrence of breast cancer. The incision had not healed though there had been ample time; this was a sign cancer was present. Dr. Thomas suggested a biopsy be performed tomorrow morning. I contacted Michael and shared my disappointing news. I explained I needed him to accompany me to the hospital. He told me not to worry and said he would make the necessary arrangements to have the day off.

It was difficult not to panic. All I could think about were the biopsies and the countless x-rays that had been performed over the last two years, all negative. On April 5, 2001, I had been diagnosed as cancer free. I refused to believe I was experiencing a recurrence of breast cancer at this stage in my life. I had done everything correctly for the past four and a half years. I had kept all my appointments and had had blood drawn, although I cried. After two years of being adamant about a recurrence of breast cancer and being told all was fine, I was devastated.

That night, Michael and I prayed fervently. We asked God to give us the courage to be strong. If we ever needed God in our lives, that was surely the time. I was terrified of the possibility of death becoming the outcome.

On the morning of my biopsy, I awakened to find out my menstrual cycle had begun. I have always experienced debilitating cramps and have taken pain medication to provide relief. The pain medication recommended eating before taking it, so I drank a quarter cup of milk and ate a half slice of bread and thought nothing of it. The food was required to prevent becoming nauseated.

We arrived at the hospital at 7:00a.m. the next morning. I did my regular routine, registered, went to my usual room, and prepared for surgery. The nurse entered my room and inquired if I had eaten or drank anything today. I replied by saying yes. She asked what I had eaten.

I said I had drunk a quarter cup of milk and had eaten a half slice of bread. The expression on her face was alarming. She excused herself and immediately left the room.

Several minutes later, Dr. Thomas entered the room and asked the same questions. I explained that I had taken medication for my menstrual cycle and that it recommend eating before taking the medication to avoid nausea. He waited patiently as I explained the instructions, and then he explained the serious reactions the milk could have with the general anesthetic. He stated that the anesthesia and milk together could cause bacteria to develop and could be fatal.

First, I thought he was kidding until I noticed the somber expression upon his face. He said if I had drunk something clear like 7-UP or Sprite, it would have been all right, but milk was not.

He said I had two options: either reschedule the biopsy or have local anesthesia and be awake during the biopsy. I chose the local.

Dr. Thomas told me the team would be down shortly. Trust me; I had no idea what was about to occur.

The team entered my room and introduced themselves. I asked everyone how the day was going. Everyone said it was going well. They began to roll my bed down the hallway. On the way to surgery, I noticed equipment and instruments in the hallway I had never seen before. Everything was all so fascinating. I was talking and having a wonderful time, as if I was on a fieldtrip.

This was my first opportunity to experience just how cold the operating rooms are. There were many different kinds of hoses and lights coming out of the ceiling. The OR reminded me of a horror movie.

Dr. Thomas finally entered the operating room and began to discuss the procedure. He said he was ready to administer the local anesthesia. A blue sheet covered my breast area, so I could not see the procedure being performed. I still had no idea what was about to happen. Then, from out of nowhere there appeared an enormous needle to be inserted into my breast. I will always remember the moment when the needle entered my breast. My legs went straight into the air. All I could do was call Dr. Thomas's name.

When the first incision was made, I knew it was startling news. Dr. Thomas's voice changed. He asked if he could take another biopsy. I asked if the cancer had returned, and he replied by saying yes and told me not to worry. Once the biopsies were completed, he mentioned he was scheduled for vacation the following day and would see me in two weeks. After we finished talking, I was immediately taken to recovery, where Michael was waiting.

Dr. Thomas met Michael and me in the recovery room. He explained I was experiencing a recurrence of breast cancer. He mentioned he had spoken with his nurse regarding ordering tests to determine the stage of cancer. She would call me later with the appointment information for a bone scan and CT scans. From the look on Michael's face, I could see he was devastated by the bewildering news.

I remained in recovery for an hour and was then discharged. On the way home, it seemed like an eternity; the drive appeared to be longer than usual. Neither Michael nor I knew how this day was going to change our lives forever. All I could do was think about the expression on Dr. Thomas's face when he performed the first biopsy.

Michael did his best to comfort me, but nothing helped the situation. During those years when I suspected a recurrence of breast cancer, I had been right. I was dumbfounded that the cancer was never detected during the previous biopsies. I struggled with the possibility that the pathology reports were never read or were not taken seriously.

When we arrived home, the nurse called regarding the appointments scheduled for the next day. I could tell from the urgency in her voice the situation was worse than I had imagined.

I was determined to remain positive. In order to have the bone and CT scans, I needed to drink a caulk-like solution and have nuclear medicine injected into my veins. This method would cause the areas where the cancer was present to light up the x-rays.

It was unnerving for me to be facing this disastrous situation. I wondered if I had the strength and courage to handle the recurrence at this point in my life. For these last several months, I had built my hopes upon the pretense I was cancer free. I had thought that in six months I would have been cancer free for five years, which is the ultimate goal in any cancer survivor's life. What could have possibly gone wrong and why? How did this silent beast within reenter my life without anyone's knowledge? Where did it come from, and where had it been concealing itself until now? Nothing made sense. One would assume that by following his or her doctor's advice, everything would be fine. Instead, my results contradicted my prognosis.

Nothing could have prepared me for the shocking information that was about to be revealed. I went to my appointment alone, thinking I could handle the diagnosis from the test results. As I sat impatiently in the examining room, listening to Dr. Thomas flipping through my bone scans and CT scan x-rays under the light, I was extremely nervous. He finally opened the door and asked if I wanted to review my x-rays. I jumped up from the examining table, still assuming the situation was not critical.

When I reviewed my x-rays, I was shaken and filled with disbelief. Not only was I experiencing a recurrence of breast cancer, but it had also metastasized to my bones. The cancer had spread to my sternum (breast bone) and other areas of my chest. I was devastated, because for four and a half years I had done all the right things. During that period, I had requested two biopsies, the first in 1999 and the second during the year 2000, because of the suspicious mass I had discovered. I had also questioned Dr. Crane numerous times regarding my medical reports. I expressed the possibility the biopsies had indicated there was a potential problem years ago.

I had trusted my life to the medical profession, and it had failed me tremendously. All I could do was cry. I knew this time for certain I was going to die in a matter of months. The breast cancer had infiltrated such a massive area of my chest; I felt the only thing to do was make funeral arrangements and notify my family and friends with the date and time.

When I called Michael, I was hysterical. I cried all the way home, wondering how this could have happened. I felt betrayed by my doctor. Apparently she never took my concerns seriously.

On the bone scan, my sternum was black, and it appeared as if I were wearing a man's necktie. The ribs attached directly to the sternum were black. I could not conceive how this devastation could have occurred, considering how much caution I had taken to stay abreast of my health.

To make matters worse, April 5, 2001, had been the last day of business for the cancer center where I had been treated. All the patients had been transferred to another cancer center because of the lack of doctors at my regular clinic. All I could think about was getting in touch with Dr. Crane. I was certain she had the answers to my questions.

Michael met me at home later. I thanked God for blessing me with this wonderful man who remained by my side all these years. I needed a rock in my life, and he was there. By then I had called Dr. Crane and explained I was experiencing a breast cancer recurrence. I inquired how I could have been cancer free in April 2001 when in July 2001 my entire chest was consumed with cancer.

Dr. Crane did not want to discuss the matter. She claimed this was a new occurrence of breast cancer. I refused to believe this was a new cancer. How could a new cancer have metastasized this quickly? And if this was a new cancer, I was in grim trouble, because at the rate it was spreading, my entire body would be consumed in a matter of months.

I was highly disappointed in her and felt she had taken the biopsy pathology reports for granted. I had thought over the years we had established a relationship in which I could contact her and discuss my medical history. Well, she had just proven me wrong. I called the medical records department and requested all of my records. I wanted to review every follow-up that had occurred over the last four and a half years. There had to be answers in my records, and I was determined to find them.

That night I prayed and pleaded with God to give me a second chance. I wasn't ready to die; I was just beginning to live and had so much life to experience. I prayed all night for God to spare my life. I promised Him if He did, I would do His will. I cried like a newborn baby coming into the world for the very first time.

During my next appointment with Dr. Thomas, I asked if he could possibly perform the surgery. He said, "Absolutely not," because of the complications and risks that were involved. He explained I needed a skillful surgeon to perform the operation. He asked us to trust him; he knew a surgeon that could perform such a delicate operation. He stated that Dr. Walker was considered to be one of the top surgeons in the field of oncology.

The following week, Michael and I met with Dr. Gaylord Walker. He looked as if he could have been on the cover of GQ magazine. We discussed the possibility of him performing the operation. He reviewed the bone and CT scans and explained the risks and complications involved.

When Dr. Walker began to discuss in detail the surgical procedures, I was dumbfounded. He said three quarters of my sternum (breastbone) needed to be removed. My ribs would be cut back; the breast reduction and implant would have to be removed because of the infiltration of the cancer. I remember asking how my body would continue to support itself if those major bones were to be removed. He laughed and reminded me the spine and shoulders are what support the body.

We discussed a tentative date for the operation. Dr. Walker knew I wanted the surgery to be performed the following day if at all possible. He said we needed to establish a trusting relationship first.

He wanted all three of us to be in agreement. I had to respect him for his logical decision, so we decided August 29, 2001, would be the day of the surgery.

When we arrived home, I immediately called and shared the devastating news regarding the surgery with my mother. Her retirement was a blessing, because she could stay as long as I needed her. My four-year-old great-nephew, Antonio, would accompany her.

He stayed with her five days a week in the suburbs to attend preschool and returned to the city on the weekend. They would be traveling with a friend from Chicago who had a daughter living in Mobile. They planned to arrive several days before the surgery.

I informed my new employer regarding my surgery and also informed him I had no idea if or when I would be retuning. This was a disheartening time in my life. I had worked extremely hard to become a successful decorator; now my dreams were being shattered, and my future did not look promising. The only thing I could do was turn my life over to the Lord. That night I thanked God for delivering me to a qualified surgeon.

I was finally at peace within and knew everything would be all right. I felt honored God had chosen me as one of his favorite people, and the experience made me humble. I love God more today than ever. I was blessed to receive this wonderful gift from God at such a critical time in my life. If there is one thing I have learned over these years, it is that He answers my prayers when I call upon Him. "God is always on time to supply my needs."

It's amazing how our lives are intertwined. When we met Dr. Walker, I knew he was my guardian angel. I had put my trust in God, and He had delivered me into the hands of a qualified and skillful surgeon. Once again I was amazed at how the divine spirit had entered our lives. God is truly amazing.

The day before surgery, Helen had relocated to Baton Rouge, Louisiana and had come down to lend moral support. Her actions touched my heart and soul. The following morning, everyone met at the hospital, and we did some serious praying. Without any doubt, this would be the lengthiest surgery I had ever endured: three hours. As usual, I requested to meet with the surgical team to reassure myself everyone was on one accord. They found it to be quite humorous, but they understood my concerns. This time my prayers were to guide the surgeon's skillful hands and spare my life.

After prayer, the team returned to take me to surgery. I kissed Michael and my mother goodbye and told the rest of my family I would see them soon. I assumed that in four to five hours I would be conscious and back to my normal self. The team and I spoke briefly until I drifted into unconsciousness.

When I awoke, it was midnight, and I immediately knew something was seriously wrong. I was in intensive care with several IVs connected to a port in my neck. There were four drainage bottles extended from side to side and in the middle of my stomach.

I panicked and called the nurse! When he arrived I asked him what was going on. He explained that the surgery had exceeded the allocated time and that I had lost a significant amount of blood, but he told me my condition was improving.

The following morning, I was delighted to see Michael and my mother. Michael explained the surgery had taken longer than anticipated because of the many complications the surgical team encountered during the surgery. When Dr. Walker entered my chest cavity, he found it was worse than anyone could have imagined. Michael also informed me that Dr. Thomas was in surgery the entire time. I told him that was impossible. He reassured me Dr. Thomas was there. I also learned my best friend Bernita and my goddaughter, Deirdre, were there during the entire surgery. She never once mentioned they would be there. It's a wonderful feeling to experience love.

I remained in the ICU (intensive care unit) for three days before I was moved to a private room. During the move, I noticed a nurse who was constantly watching me, making me feel uncomfortable.

She finally approached me and asked if I was Brenda Rocker. I did not answer her immediately, so she repeated herself. I finally answered her, and that's when she stated that when they brought me out of surgery, I had lost such a substantial amount of blood that I was unrecognizable and looked like a white blob. At first it was difficult for me to comprehend what she meant. Although my skin is fair, my features are prominent. There is no mistake I'm an African-American. There was only one explanation; the substantial blood loss had drained all the color from my skin.

The joy of knowing God was with me during such a critical time in surgery left me experiencing total peace within. Apparently at one time it must have appeared to be a touch-and-go situation. I knew for certain that if it had not been for God, I would not have survived the complications from surgery. By His grace alone I was spared! It's an awesome feeling to be a recipient of God's love.

Later that night I began hallucinating from the morphine. The morphine was being administered through the PC (pain control) machine through an IV, making me feel as though I was dreaming.

The hallucinations were of giant children wearing athletic outfits, playing basketball and holding me hostage in their home. Each time I tried to escape, one of them would catch me and cover me with enormous sofa cushions. The hallucinations lasted for several hours at a time.

Once I was able to stay awake for an hour, and then I dozed off again.

This time I began to hallucinate about the windows revolving around the room; I tried to catch them, only to have them slip through my hands each time. I became frightened and called the nurse on duty.

When she arrived, I shared my frightening experiences with her and asked her to please remove the morphine IV. She told me she wasn't authorized to remove the IV but would speak with the interns when they made their morning rounds.

Morning finally arrived. The hallucinations had continued throughout the night and had been a frightening experience. When the interns made their morning rounds, I asked to have the morphine IV removed. One of the interns stated I needed the morphine because of the complications that had occurred during surgery. I explained I wasn't experiencing any pain or discomfort but was only experiencing hallucinations. They finally agreed to disconnect the IV from the PC machine.

Later that day I had a very special visitor; Dr. Thomas stopped by, concerned about me. I mentioned Michael had informed me he had been in surgery with me. He said Michael was absolutely correct.

Dr. Walker had requested his presence in the operating room. He then apologized and told me that if the procedures he performed during the reconstruction surgery caused the cancer to metastasize, he was immensely sorry. I explained it was my decision to have the procedures performed.

I hoped he knew just how those words touched me. Those words remain with me until this very day. I always knew Dr. Thomas was a wonderful person and a child of God. His actions confirmed my thoughts. I was blessed. God had put this remarkable man in my life, if only for a season.

That same day, more special guests visited me from my dad's 2001 family reunion, which was in Jackson, Mississippi—a three-hour drive away. My Dad, Uncle Tommy, Aunt Lily, and my cousin Chip took the time out to drive to Mobile. My cousin Tyrone took military leave to spend time with us during my recovery. The support of family and friends was marvelous. For me, nothing is better than seeing loved ones during a recovery; it's the best medication that can possibly be prescribed.

Later that evening, Dennis from Harlem's stopped by with two beautiful floral arrangements. The floral arrangement in the crystal vase was special. Dennis and several other coworkers purchased the vase, which held a beautiful arrangement of long-stemmed yellow roses. The reason that particular arrangement was special was that I had planned to purchase the crystal vase myself. The vase was beautiful, with stunning diamond cuts in the design. The second arrangement was in a silver decanter with short red roses and was decorated just as beautifully as the first.

I had as well received several other beautiful arrangements from family and friends. I was touched by everyone's kindness and support. This was a spiritual reward I was receiving. It's during critical times in our lives that we discover who our loved ones are. They are there to provide love and the moral support that is required through difficult chapters in one's life.

I thanked God for allowing Dr. Thomas to enter my life through Dr. Crane. I know that because of his genuine love and compassion he was instrumental in saving my life. I will always be indebted to this wonderful man. His family is blessed to have this remarkable man in their lives. He is my hero and will always have a special place in my heart. I can say I love this remarkable man.

I have finally come to terms regarding Dr. Crane as well, and have realized that without her in my life, I never would have had the opportunity to meet Dr. Thomas. I have learned it was erroneous for me to have thought our relationship was more than a doctor–patient relationship. I had taken for granted that because of the time we had invested over the years, I could speak with her regarding my health at any time. I determined that in order for me to get past that horrific chapter of my life, I needed to forgive Dr. Crane for any injustice I thought she might have committed against me.

Chapter Eight:

Chest Reconstruction Surgery

I WOULD LIKE TO SHARE my medical records from July 30, 2001 through August 29, 2001. The medical records consist of the biopsy and chest reconstruction. I'm sure everyone will be amazed as to what will be revealed.

PATIENT: Rocker, Brenda
CHART: 58011-8
DATE: 7-30-01

Mrs. Rocker is present today after having fallen when climbing up on her refrigerator approximately three months ago. She sustained some sort of abrasion or tear of the left medial breast just adjacent to the area of incision from the previous reduction mammoplasty. This has not fully healed over the course of follow-up. There is some skin breakdown there but more concerning is a bit of mass affect around here. I'm not sure if this represents some form of chronic infection versus neoplasia. I have advised biopsy of this area. The biopsy was scheduled. Outpatient H & P was done and handwritten and documented. Questions were answered fully. Informed consent was given.

Patient: ROCKER, BRENDA E
MR# 20146829
Admit: 08/01/2001
Attending Physician:
Patient Type: O
Room #
Age: 43Y Sex: F

OPERATIVE REPORT
DATE OF SURGERY: 8/01/01
SURGEON: ASSISTANT DR:
PREOPERATIVE DIAGNOSIS: LEFT BREAST MASS
OPERATION: EXCISIONAL BIOPSY OF
LEFT BREAST MASS AND
EXCORIATION

INDICATIONS: The patient is a 43-year old lady with a previous history of breast cancer who has undergone breast reconstruction.

She developed an area of excoriation on the medial side of the left mastectomy reduction site where she fell on her refrigerator several months ago. This has not healed over. There was an area of mass effect beneath that, and this was fairly close and intimately related to the previous right mastectomy scar from the breast cancer treatment.

At any rate, as this had not healed over, I felt biopsy was warranted.

The risks for further surgery, bleeding, infection, pregnancy, etc., were all discussed. Informed consent was given.

DESCRIPTION OF PROCEDURE: After written permission was secured, the patient was brought to surgery, where satisfactory mask sedation was achieved. The usual sterile prep and drape was done.

An ellipse was designed around the nodular area in question where the non- healing area of skin excoriation was. Approximately

2" was outlined for the elliptical excision. Xylocaine with epinephrine solution was infiltrated and a field block was applied.

The resection was done. There appeared to be quite abnormal tissue deep within. It was submitted for pathology. A culture was taken. Hemostasis was meticulous.

Layered wound closure was affected. A dressing was applied and the procedure was terminated. The patient was taken from surgery in satisfactory condition.

END OF REPORT

CHART: 11111111
DATE: 8/13/01

Mrs. Rocker is present today for discussion following the CT examination, bone scan etc. The bone scan lights up on the sternum and on the CT scan I can see what looks to be tumorous involvement extending from the right side over and this appears to involve the area of the sternum bone there. I have therefore advised consultation with Dr. Walker, a surgical oncologist, for consideration of chest wall resection. I have explained to Mrs. Rocker that this is certainly a very large operation and will carry significant risks. Copies of her records were made for Dr. Walker review along with the path report and she is going to transports the x-rays over.

END OF REPORT

CENTER FOR PLASTIC AND RECONSTRUCTIVE SURGERY
AND CENTER FOR HAND SURGERY
August 13, 2001
RE: Brenda Rocker
DOB 3-25-58

Dear Dr. Walker

I saw Mrs. Rocker back in the office August 13, 2001. As
we discussed by telephone, she appears to have sternum
involvement with recurrent breast cancer from her previous right breast cancer.

This does extend over the midline somewhat. She will be
transporting

CT scan and bone scan for your review. I hope that you
can assist with this difficult problem. Please don't hesitate
to let me know if I may assist in any way.

Sincerely,

Dr. Thomas
Division of Plastic and Reconstructive
Surgery

END OF REPORT

BRENDA E. ROCKER
MRN:
H#
DOB: 03/25 /1958 AGE: 43 YRS
RM/BED:
COPY TO:
LOCATION:

SURGICAL PATHOLOGY REPORT
COMMENT:

The resected portion of sternum includes overlying skin and soft tissue on the left side of the specimen identified by the surgeon as tissue that was continuous with the medial edge of the resected left breast. This soft tissue contains a 3.0 cm nodule of carcinoma. This carcinoma, then could have arisen in the very medial portion of the breast, or may be a metastasis in the soft tissue immediately medial to the left breast. No breast parenchyma is identified in the tissue around this 3.0 cm nodule. The carcinoma extends the periosteum of the sternum.

Multiple sections of the sternum reveal a separate focus of carcinoma at the right, superior edge of the specimen. This focus wasn't apparent grossly and measures only 0.3 cm. Its presence is immediately adjacent to the cartilage and does extend to the inked surgical margin.

The patient has a history of infiltration ductal carcinoma in the right breast for which she underwent mastectomy 1997. That procedure was performed elsewhere, and the slides were reviewed here in 1997 (85 -3685). The slides were subsequently returned, but the review revealed that the right breast cancer extended into the skeletal muscle, and 1 of 18 right axillary lymph nodes contained metastatic cancer.

END OF REPORT

PATIENT: ROCKER, BRENDA
MNN:
H#:
DOB: 03/251958 AGE: 43 YRS
RM/BED
COPY TO:
LOCATION:
SURGICAL PATHOLOGY REPORT
ACCESSION DATE: 08/29/01
COMMENT:

The 3.0 cm nodule of carcinoma in the soft tissue over the left side of the sternum then could represent either a new, left breast primary lesion or chest wall recurrence of the right breast cancer. Given that a separate, grossly undetectable, 0.3 cm nodule of similar carcinoma was identified adjacent to cartilage along the right superior sternum and that no breast parenchyma was histologically evident adjacent to the 3.0 cm focus suggests that both of these lesion could represent recurrence of the right breast carcinoma.

The 3.0 cm nodule of carcinoma closely approached but is not seen to involve the surgical margin. The 0.3 cm focus of carcinoma extends to the inked surgical margin.

The findings were discussed with Dr. Thomas

By: Dr. Walker

Chapter Nine:

Coping With Disabilities

I WAS DISCHARGED FROM THE hospital September 3, 2001. When I arrived home, my first request was to view my incision. Michael undressed me carefully. Once the bandages were completely off, I realized the significance of my surgery. My incision extended from my right armpit to my left armpit. I had four Jackson-Pratt drainage bottles, two located on each side of my body and two in the middle of my stomach. There were over a hundred stitches holding the incision together.

This was the first time I welcomed this sight, because my life had been saved by this delicate operation I had endured. While lying in bed, trying to recuperate and put the past behind me, I couldn't help but wonder how this situation had escalated to this level. I was just as baffled as everyone else regarding the breast cancer recurrence.

I thanked God for giving me another chance at life. I had spent the last several years trying to convince my doctors there was a potential crisis involving a recurrence. Everyone was in awe regarding why the two biopsies performed in the year 1999 and in the year 2000 never revealed the cancer. My thoughts are that the pathology reports were either never read or not read properly. I always felt there was a reason to be alarmed, and now I regret not following my mind and getting a second medical opinion.

I know God led me to our house and made it possible for us to close in less than thirty days. My unfortunate accident saved my life. If it had not been for us moving, chances are I would have never injured my breast, and the recurrence would have been discovered after my death, during the autopsy. I looked upon our home as a blessing from God; it will always have an extraordinary place in my heart.

I'm also aware my life is a gift from God and can be taken in an instant. This is why we should live our lives as if each day is our last day on earth; only then can we appreciate the gift of life. You never realize how precious life is until it is taken away.

I was blessed to have my mother with me during such a critical time in my life. Her presence was truly comforting. I knew this time I needed her to stay the entire month because of the seriousness of the surgery. I found it difficult moving about with the four Jackson-Pratt drainage bottles, which caused pain and discomfort each time I moved. I also discovered I could no longer lie on my stomach because of the extreme pressure caused by the removal of the sternum.

It's impossible for me to rest comfortably. And I anticipated the day when the drainage bottles would be removed and my sternum would heal.

After I was up and about, Antonio asked me if I could turn the ceiling fan off in the bedroom. The only way I could reach the fan was to stand in the bed. Although I was able to get onto the bed, I was unable to get off. After discovering that I couldn't bend down, Antonio realized I was in trouble and ran for Michael's assistance.

It's amazing how I once took simple body movements for granted. Just a month before I could have performed that task in less than a second. Now I find myself wishing I could change my past and make things the way they were. Life is full of uncertainties, and you never know when your life may experience a drastic change. This why I now treasure every waking moment.

The most valuable lesson I have learned is that my loved ones mean the world to me and that I would be in total despair without them. Our loved ones are irreplaceable; when they are gone, there is no coming back, and we are left with only memories to cherish.

Today I had the Jackson-Pratt drainage bottles removed. This time, instead of having two drainage bottles removed, there were four. When Dr. Walker began to remove the first one, my memories of 1997 resurfaced. I did not know how I would survive this terrible ordeal. Each time he removed a drainage bottle;

I grabbed hold of his lab coat and screamed. When the last drainage bottle was removed, I was overcome with joy.

I also spoke with Dr. Thomas and Dr. Walker concerning my recovery. They both informed me it would take at least five years before my body began to recover from the surgery. I knew I needed to make adjustments in my life but prayed my recovery would be speedier than what had been forecasted. I had already started my arm therapy of walking the walls to prevent "cold shoulder." I knew the therapy would be more difficult because of the four drainage bottles restricting my movement.

With limitations in my life, I knew I would be restricted from doing simple things like cooking and cleaning. Being totally dependent upon my family was the most difficult adjustment to make. I have always prided myself on being self-reliant. I was determined that in six months my body would recover by at least 70%. Each day, I tried to increase my activities, but I was careful not to overexert myself and cause a setback in my recovery.

Today I have accepted my disability and fully understand I am unable to work. At the time, I was aware I needed a reliable source of income. So, I decided to go to the Social Security Administration office. There I inquired about the possibilities of drawing Social Security benefits but was informed that qualifying for Supplemental Security Income (SSI) would be difficult. My attitude remained positive, and I felt whatever happened will be for the best. The caseworker I spoke with was compassionate. He said he would do everything within his power to get my benefits approved. I thanked him for his assistance and went on my way.

Once leaving the Social Security office, I decided that since I was already out, I would go to the specialty shop which was located at Memorial Hospital. I needed to have my breast prosthesis fitted.

There was a variety of styles of prostheses to choose from, as well as an assortment of bras. They were available in black, beige, and white, and they were decorated with lace trimming. The fitting was performed by a specialist named Yvonne. She took her time as she made all the proper adjustments to ensure that both breast prostheses and bras fit correctly and comfortably.

The month passed quickly, and it was time for my mother and nephew to return home. I knew I would miss Antonio; he was a tremendous helper although he was only four years of age. He tried to clean the bathroom once because, as he said, "Uncle Michael sure does get the floor wet when he showers."

Antonio checked on me throughout the day to make sure I had plenty of ice in my cup. He was unaware that I could see him in the hallway when he took a few pieces of the ice before he entered the room. I received pleasure in watching him.

In the morning, Bernita and Deirdre were taking my mother and Antonio to the Greyhound bus station. I was relieved they were taking the bus and not flying, because of the recent terrorists attacks that had occurred in New York and Washington. My mother would rather take the long ride and feel safe. Their presence would be missed immensely in our home.

My godmother, Alice (Faye), would be driving down from Joliet, Illinois in a few days to assist me for a couple of weeks. We met over thirty years ago, and she remains a positive role model in my life. I impatiently awaited her arrival; I just wished it could be under different circumstances.

I hoped we would be able to take in a movie. And this opportunity would give us a chance to catch up on what's been happening in our families' lives. Although, we had not seen each other in several years, we talked frequently on the telephone. I had recently made her a beautiful leopard-print comforter with matching pillows from my design label, Creative Concepts. The comforters are handcrafted using quality fabrics, and plenty of love and commitment goes into the finished product.

I was excited to see Faye. She looked fantastic! I love her like a mother. Faye welcomed me into her home when I was fifteen years of age. At the time, her three young children were ten, seven, and four years of age. And her children respect me as their oldest sister. There is an enormous amount of love and history in our lives, and it's an honor and a privilege to have her in our home. Her conversations are always positive and encouraging. She makes everyone she encounters feel special. I love her and feel blessed having her in my life.

Once Faye was settled in, we decided to go to the mall for a outing, and I learned the hard way that my body had not begun to recover. I could not walk a quarter of the mall; the reality was I could not accept the fact I was unable to do simple things. I also discovered while out that if I was out of bed for more than a couple of hours, an immense amount of pressure built up in my chest. I became exhausted quickly; Faye understood and suggested I try to take it easy.

The following week, Faye and I were at the clinic for my oncology checkup. Everything went well, and my body was healing as predicted. My next appointment, and evaluation, was scheduled for one month later. I hoped I would be well enough to drive myself to my appointment.

When we arrived home, Faye began to pack for her trip home. We enjoyed the rest of the evening, talking and reminiscing about the good old days. Later Faye turned in early to bed so she could get an early start in the morning.

For my first appointment at Central hospital cancer center, I was immediately disenchanted with the operation. There were about thirty patients all crammed into a small waiting area. I could sense everyone was uncomfortable with the situation. There were some deathly ill patients grouped with other cancer patients that were not as critical. Cancer is an illness not everyone can handle, and some people prefer to be isolated from others.

I was sitting across from a patient who looked as if she could die any day. Her entire body was wrapped in a strange garment. Never before had I seen anything like it. She had IVs in one of her hands and in her neck. Her facial expression informed us that she was suffering and was in an enormous amount of pain. She should have been in a private examining room, lying down. On the other side of me sat a man who could barely move. Emotionally, I couldn't handle this situation. I looked perfectly healthy and was sure some people were wondering why I was there.

Once my name was called, I thought I was being taken to a private examining room. I soon learned that wasn't the case. There was a nurse drawing blood while six of us waited in one room as we watched each patient having his or her blood drawn. Because of the removal of the lymph nodes from underneath both my arms, my blood could only be drawn from my feet at that time. Just because I was watching everyone, I suffered an anxiety attack and felt as if I was about to faint.

When it was my turn to have my blood drawn, I informed the nurse I emotionally couldn't handle it. She realized the situation could change at any moment, and not for the better. The nurse stated they would wait and draw my blood on my next appointment. My name was called again, and I was finally taken to an examining room. There I waited forty-five minutes for the doctor. I couldn't comprehend what was happening; everything seemed chaotic.

While waiting in the examining room, I quickly noticed there were no medical degrees or licenses hanging on the wall. The only items indicating this was an examining room were an examining table and chair. The room had a cold and impersonal feeling. I was never given a gown to wear for the examination. I had made up my mind that if I waited five more minutes I would leave and locate an oncologist myself.

Dr. Scott entered the room, and appeared to be distraught. I could see she had been bombarded by patients all day. She asked routine questions and wanted to know how I had been doing since my surgery. I informed her I was not experiencing any complications from the surgery. Dr. Scott did a quick examination with my blouse open and instructed me to make an appointment to see her in three months.

Before I left, I questioned her regarding her medical degrees and licenses for the state of Alabama. She replied by telling me she had just recently graduated from the School of Oncology in New Orleans and had been practicing medicine there for many years as well. I asked her if her medical degrees and licenses would be posted in a conspicuous place when I returned. She said yes, so I took her word and scheduled the appointment for three months later.

Perhaps I may have been a bit judgmental about the situation, but I was used to organization and privacy. I felt the situation should have been better organized, considering the cancer center had been operating since the end of April and it was September. Perhaps instead of transferring all the cancer patients to one clinic, we should have been split up into smaller groups and referred to local clinics that could better accommodate the influx of new cancer patients.

Before leaving the hospital, I stopped by the medical records department to inform the staff I would be returning to pick up copies of my records for my review at a later date. That way, if I had any questions regarding my treatment, I could always refer to the medical documents. The nurse questioned me as to why I needed my medical records. I explained to her that I kept copies of my medical records at home. By law, I'm entitled to copies of my medical records at my request, even if there is a fee involved.

I left the clinic concerned regarding the medical care I had received. I hated myself for being so critical and judgmental, but first impressions do have a significant impact in any situation.

However, I needed to realize that not all environments I encountered would be as well organized as my own surroundings. I tried to be understanding and gave them the benefit of the doubt; I thought perhaps it was just a difficult day they were experiencing. All along, I was hoping this wasn't the normal operation of the business.

When Michael returned home, I informed him of the insufficient healthcare I had experienced. He asked if I was aware of any other alternatives for treatment. I mentioned I would see Dr. Walker before my next appointment and discuss my concerns. I just wanted a doctor who was competent and had my best interests at heart. Unfortunately, I had already experienced inadequate healthcare, and as a result it almost cost me my life.

Because of my apprehensiveness regarding the cancer center, I couldn't help wondering if, during my treatment there (if I chose to continue with it) I would have peace of mind or would always be skeptical of the medical treatment I had received. One thing is for certain: I cannot handle being in a crowded waiting room. In my opinion, I deserve to be treated with respect and dignity. For me, that requires privacy.

During my oncology checkup with Dr. Walker, I expressed my concerns regarding the healthcare I had received and asked if there was another facility at which I could receive treatments. I mentioned I was contemplating seeking medical care elsewhere. He said he understood my concerns, but he said that on my next visit the situation might improve, so I decided to give Dr. Scott another try. Before leaving the clinic, I stopped by the records department to retrieve my medical records from the previous appointment. The clerk again inquired as to why I needed copies of the records. I explained that I maintained copies of my medical records for future reference.

Sometimes when I was reviewing my records, I found statements and comments transcribed that were never mentioned during my appointments. I always wrote information down regarding any concerns or questions I might have.

I'm sure most people might say I'm paranoid, and they are absolutely correct. We only get one life, and once it's gone, that's it. Regardless of all the apologies in the world, nothing can bring you back. We forget that we pay our doctors' salaries and that we have the right to voice our opinions and concerns regarding our healthcare, Remember, we have the right to choose another healthcare provider; just remember who is paying whom!

When I arrived home, I received excellent news from the Social Security Administration: my benefits had been approved. The monthly benefits were more than I had anticipated. That's when I learned there are two Social Security benefit programs that are available.

There is Supplemental Security Income, which is better known as SSI, and there is Social Security Disability Insurance which is known as SSDI. I would receive SSDI because I had always worked and had paid enough money into Social Security. This qualifies me for my Social Security benefits. A percentage of my earnings over the years of employment determine my monthly benefits.

Now, there is a twist to this magnificent news. I could not draw my SSDI until I had been disabled for five months, and unlike SSI, there was no back-pay involved. I wondered if the administration anticipated my death within those five months and whether the benefits would roll over into another account or program if this was the case.

In any case, it was critical that I manage my savings for the following five months in order to meet my monthly obligations. My first disability check was scheduled to arrive in March 2002, around my birthday. The check would be considered a gift from God.

Until I received my first benefit check, I would remain pessimistic about my approval. I felt that any day someone would phone and say, "We are sorry; a mistake was made regarding your SSDI and your benefits have been denied. Please schedule another appointment."

I decided to celebrate my birthday in March with a festive celebration with one hundred guests. We would have a marvelous time entertaining family and friends as they enjoyed delicious food and spirits. Their presence would be the greatest gift I could ever receive. I had five months to plan for the event and make it a memorable and joyous occasion. This would be a spectacular time in my life.

I also became more comfortable with my body. My new scars represented life, and I would not trade them for anything in the world. I had also started dressing and undressing in front of Michael again; I had come to the realization, that if he loved me before the surgery he loved me after the surgery. The only difference was that I no longer had breasts; I had been set free of my inhibitions!

I had my second appointment with Dr. Scott and had ample time to asses the operation of the cancer center. I remained adamant about not receiving chemotherapy; however, I decided to take the cancer-blocker pill; the side effects had been drastically reduced. I would also take a cancer-blocker injection, which was supposed to increase the chances of the cancer going into remission. After my evaluation, Dr. Scott determined the next day would be the perfect time to have the injection, because my cycle had recently ended. The injections were to be administered in the buttock. I hoped to do well with these two methods of treatment.

The following morning, I got dressed and was out of the house by 7:00 a.m. My appointment was scheduled for 8:00 a.m., and I wanted to be prepared to sign and fill out any necessary documents for the injection. The nurse at the front desk was courteous and handed me a clipboard with an application and consent forms to fill out. Once I had completed the forms, I returned them to her and took a seat. After sitting down, I noticed how beautifully the waiting area had been decorated with an array of various shades of blue.

The nurse administering the injection called my name and escorted me to an examining room. There was a hospital bed along with an oxygen tank. I was apprehensive but decided not to say a word. The nurse instructed me to sit on the bed as she prepared the injection. I waited patiently as she finished her preparation. Then she instructed me to lie on my back and to lift up my blouse. That's when I questioned her; she explained the injection was to be administered to my abdomen. She apologized for me being misinformed.

I explained to her I wasn't emotionally prepared for the injection to be administered to my abdomen I informed her regarding my phobia of needles. She was patient and said she understood.

I requested to see the needle; that was a big mistake! The needle held a small pellet that was to be injected below my navel. Tears began to roll down my face.

I called Michael and explained the situation to him. He said he would meet me at the hospital. When I hung up the phone, I realized that by the time Michael arrived, the injection could be over. I called him back and requested he not come; then I told the nurse to proceed with the injection. Once the pellet entered my body, it burned like hell, and it was difficult to regain my composure. I couldn't wait for my next oncology checkup with Dr. Scott to tell her she had misinformed me about the procedure.

It distressed me to learn some doctors do not research new medications before recommending them to their patients. I am positive doctors receive literature on new medications and procedures before they are available to their patients. I understood at that point why careless mistakes were made in the medical profession. If doctors and their staff members were more knowledgeable about new procedures and medications, it could possibly eliminate some of the malpractice suits. This causes their insurance rates to increase, thereby passing the cost onto their patients.

Now I understand why some people do not seek medical assistance out of fear. They don't trust the doctors, and without trust people cannot build a relationship. Patients need to know their doctors are there to provide them with quality healthcare. When we leave the hospital, one should be confident regarding the recommendations of treatments and prescribed medications by his or her physician.

In March 2002, I received my Social Security benefits check. Now that I was officially on a fixed income, I realized I needed to eliminate luxury items that were not necessities. I realized I needed to limit my spending if I expected to survive from month to month. This would be a difficult adjustment. When I was earning an excellent income, not once did I ever have a second thought about how carelessly I spent my money. If I saw something that I liked, I would purchase it.

That evening, we would celebrate my birthday, and I expected an excellent turnout. I had prepared plenty of delicious food. Some of the dishes had taken several days to prepare. Family and friends from out of town were arriving to help celebrate this magnificent occasion in my life. My dad and Uncle Roosevelt drove from Chicago but would be leaving before the party. They had a previous engagement Sunday evening.

My dad and I picked up my birthday cake. We had no idea how enormous it would be. The cake was large enough to serve over one hundred people—depending upon the size of the slices, of course. The only way to transport the cake home was for me to sit in the back seat and hold it. The cake was decorated very beautifully and outlined in red roses.

The icing, which is my favorite part of the cake, was butter cream. The menu consisted of chicken baked in a hot salsa, swedish meatballs, ham, turkey, crab salad, quiche, potato salad, pasta salad, three-bean salad, fresh fruit, and dinner rolls. I felt confident there was something to satisfy everyone's appetite; the guests would be discussing how spectacular and delicious everything was for days to come.

The excitement was building inside of me; I could not wait for the party to begin. This was going to be my best birthday celebration ever. That night, I would greet my guests while wearing a navy gown with sequins and silver evening shoes; I wanted to feel glamorous, although my guests would be dressed casually. The house was decorated beautifully, the table was set in linen, and fresh flowers were everywhere. The food presentation was awesome! There was enough food to feed over one hundred guests, and I hoped everyone attending the celebration would be enthusiastic and in good spirits!

The guests began to arrive, and it looked like a terrific turnout.

I was glad I had decided to decorate the patio. There were numerous people outdoors, enjoying the weather. Although it was the end of March, the temperature was in the '60s. Everyone who came brought me a gift. It felt like I was celebrating my twenty-first birthday. Everyone loved how beautifully everything was decorated.

I was touched by the number of the people who came out to celebrate my forty-fourth birthday. Receiving all the hugs, kisses, and gifts made me feel like a queen, and I enjoyed every moment of the attention I received. Without a doubt, I knew it was absolutely a blessing from God for me to be there, celebrating my life.

After the guests sang "Happy Birthday to You," I cried tears of joy and began to open my gifts. I received an abundance of wonderful gifts, including miniature figurines. How amazed I was to learn that so many of my acquaintances knew my desires. Everything was marvelous, and the celebration ended around 2:30 a.m. That night will always represent a memorable occasion in my heart.

Chapter Ten:

Adjusting to Life's Changes

I FOUND IT EXTREMELY DIFFICULT adjusting to many of life's changes. Simple tasks I once took for granted, I found to be difficult. I became exhausted just from a walk through my house and it was difficult to sit up for one or two hours consecutively. This situation had occurred because of the disconnection of the sternum and ribs. Because of this, my ribs were constantly moving, appearing to float. The moving caused a significance amount of discomfort. And, because a major portion of my sternum had been removed, I could see my heart beating through my skin.

A significant amount of time had passed since my last appointment with Dr. Scott. I reached the conclusion she was bombarded with far too many patients, so I decided to see Dr. Walker for my oncology checkups. There were several reasons for my decision.

The first was the lack of knowledge regarding the injections, for which I paid dearly. Over time, the injection causes the vagina to lose its natural lubricants, which causes irritation. Apparently those side effects were never taken into consideration. The side effects from the injections were so unbearable that sometimes I had to relieve myself by sitting in tubs of cold water. Perhaps if there had been a cream available to provide some form of relief, it would have been more tolerable. The only positive thing regarding the injections was that they put me into a temporary menopause, stopping my cycle. But once the medication from the injections was completely out of my system, my cycle resumed.

My second reason: I require quality time with my physicians. I consider myself a sound investment, and therefore I expect to have my questions answered and my concerns put to rest. I should not feel as if I am imposing on their time at any appointments.

Over time, I had forgiven Dr. Crane for contributing to my becoming disabled, but I felt the cancer center should have been liable for my inadequate healthcare. My entire life had changed drastically, so I decided to seek the advice of an attorney. I also knew the statute of limitations was running out to file a lawsuit; therefore, I needed to proceed quickly. I gathered all my medical documentation that was relevant to the case and set an appointment.

During the consultation, the attorney and I discussed the possibilities of filing a malpractice suit. He wrote down the pertinent information required for the evaluation. He explained that the law firm had a physician on staff and that based upon his finding, a decision would be made regarding a malpractice suit. The evaluation would take a week, and I would be notified for my next consultation.

The week passed quickly. On the day of my second consultation, I was dressed and out of the house by 9:00 a.m.; I wanted to be prompt. I wondered if the news would be terrific or disappointing. Either way, I would learn the outcome that day.

During the appointment the attorney informed me their doctors had determined I had received adequate medical care under Dr. Crane simply because she had ordered a chest x-ray and a mammogram, regardless of whether the radiology reports were ever read. I was baffled at this determination; although the yearly mammograms and chest x-rays were ordered, the breast cancer was undiagnosed for several years. And the two biopsies performed in the years 1999 and 2000 had no relevance, although they clearly revealed there was a problem. Both biopsies stressed the concerns of the activity in my "first lesion." At that moment I realized no one would ever learn if the pathology reports had ever been read. Accepting the outcome enabled me to close this catastrophic chapter in my life.

Over the years I have become skillful in interpreting human behavior. And I have determined the world is made up of two kinds of people: those who give and those who take. I have witnessed family and friends abandon their loved ones during critical times in their lives. Some will abandon people out of fear the person may die or may require assistance. I imagine the most earth-shattering circumstance is dying alone. Trust me; if the shoe were on the other foot, they would want their loved ones to be there to comfort them in this time of need.

Life's mishaps have a way of opening our eyes to situations that are otherwise oblivious to the human mind. I pray I will forever remain the person I am, always willing to support a loved one, a friend, or even a stranger if a crisis should occur.

I can't help but recollect an acquaintance that ended our friendship during a crisis in my life. One year later this same acquaintance became ill; I tried to ignore her when she reached out for my assistance, but I couldn't. Everyone who she thought was her friend deserted her during a heart-rending moment in her life. She quickly learned I was the only person who came to her assistance.

Everyone should experience walking in each other's shoes. By doing this we will appreciate each other and be more sympathetic and compassionate to other's emotions. We have a tendency to think life will remain the same as it was yesterday, but in the blink of an eye our lives can be turned upside down. Life can throw poignant blows, and some people never recover from them.

One day my friend Denise stopped by and shared a heartbreaking story with me. Her sister had been diagnosed with breast cancer three years before and had decided to stop taking her medication. She had been seeing an herbalist that practiced alternative medicine and was treating her with herbs. He informed her she was two years cancer free. Her condition started deteriorating soon following her prognosis. She was hospitalized and given bone and CT scans, which revealed the breast cancer had metastasized throughout her entire body. When she passed, she was in her early fifties. Chances are that if she had continued taking her medicine and had kept her regularly scheduled checkups, she might be alive today.

After listening to her heartbreaking story, I reflected back to the day of the freak accident that saved my life. God intervened in my life; He knew I had become complacent concerning my treatment.

For the first time in four and a half years, I accepted my diagnosis without questioning my oncologist. When I had my suspicions regarding the recurrence of breast cancer, I should have sought a second opinion. I trusted my instincts more since experiencing the recurrence.

I believe most people don't understand herbal medicine. Herbs can aid in the prevention of certain diseases. Regrettably, they cannot prevent a disease that already exists. If it were simple to rid the body of cancer, there would be scores of people alive today as a result of herbal therapy. Therefore, if you plan to practice herbal therapy, start now; do not wait until being diagnosed with cancer or any other disease. And if you chose herbal therapy for healing, I would recommend that you should still seek the assistance of a physician; after all, you cannot see inside of your body. Be wise and live a long and fulfilling life.

Just when I thought my day could not get any worse, Helen called and informed me of Sandy's death in Houston. She had lost her battle with breast cancer. Her departure was truly a sorrowful one, because it could have been avoided. When she realized the prayers alone were not working, she decided to have the chemotherapy, but the cancer had already metastasized throughout her entire body. She started going blind nine months prior to her death. I wondered how Sandy's male companion was handling her death. He was somewhat responsible; because of his selfishness, she tried desperately to hold on to her vanity. I was sure she would be greatly missed by her friends and loved ones.

Breast cancer is a silent killer; there are no signs or warning until it's too late. There is no pain or discomfort associated with the disease until the final stages. Within five years, this silent killer can infiltrate the body and cause devastation that's irreversible. The only way to have a fighting chance against the silent beast within is to have yearly mammograms and PET/CT scans. At the present time, these are our best weapons of defense.

I'm sure if I had not had yearly mammograms, I would have died within the first five years from the day of developing breast cancer. That is why, when I'm sharing my breast cancer experience with women, I always strongly suggest having yearly mammograms. The mammogram only takes five to ten minutes to complete. There is a little discomfort involved, but that could very well be the difference between life and death. Although there is a substantial number of women without medical insurance, they still have the opportunity to have a yearly mammogram. Also, in some states across the country, you can get a mammogram for free if you cannot afford it.

Several months ago I had developed pain in my chest, and I was confused, because my chest area should still have been numb as a result of the severed nerves. I had begun to document the pain so that I could remember to speak with Dr. Walker regarding the pain at my next checkup.

During my last visit with Dr. Walker, I informed him of the debilitating pain I had been experiencing in my chest, and he stated I should still be numb in both arms and my chest. I can recall regaining sensation in my arms in March of 2003; it felt as if currents of electricity were shooting through my body. I thought this was a natural occurrence due to the nerves' mending but Dr. Walker insisted severed nerves don't have the capability to mend, leaving no medical explanation for my discomfort.

At times when the pain was extremely intense, I called my sisters, Elaine and Kimberly. We talked for hours to distract my mind until I gained relief. Sometimes I walked the floor, crying and praying for hours for the pain to subside. Each day the pain was becoming more unbearable, so I decided to schedule an appointment with my general practitioner, Dr. White, hoping she could determine what was causing the pain. I did not know how much more of the pain I could tolerate. I also believed I have damaged my stomach lining by overdosing with the pain medication I used to treat my arthritis.

When I arrived for my appointment with Dr. White, I signed in and waited to be called. My vital signs were taken and were excellent. The nurse asked what kind of problems I was experiencing. I explained about the excruciating pain in my chest and arms. She wrote down the information and said Dr. White would be with me momentarily.

When Dr. White entered the room, she brought her beautiful smile and wonderful bedside manners as usual. When I met her, my first impression was that I was dealing with someone just out of college. She looked to be twenty years of age. She asked what was wrong, and I explained about the agonizing pain in my chest and right arm. I mentioned my stomach lining was upset because of the pain medication.

She explained the dangers of exceeding the recommended dosage of the medication and mentioned it could cause stomach ulcers and other serious complications.

Then she advised me not to take any more of the medication and prescribed two hundred milligrams of a new medication that is currently available on the market. The medication is used to treat severe arthritis without causing damage to the stomach lining. I was praying for relief from the pain and was willing to try anything. I left the clinic and drove directly to the pharmacy to have the prescription filled.

Several hours passed, and there were still no signs of relief from the medication. I walked the floor, anticipating the relief. The pain persisted for hours; then I recalled Dr. Thomas had given me a prescription several years ago for a narcotic pain medication. When I located the medication, I immediately took two pills and rested until the medication began to provide relief. Because of the chronic pain in my chest, I was in constant fear that I was experiencing a recurrence of bone cancer. And if that was the case, I feared the outcome. There were no other bones in my body that could be removed. My mind was filled with thoughts of finally succumbing to bone cancer.

As a result of my many fears of suffering another recurrence, I decided to schedule another appointment with Dr. Walker, determined to convince him I had regained sensation in my chest and both arms, regardless of medical science. After arriving for my appointment, I signed in and waited for the nurse to call me. She took my vitals signs and asked if I was experiencing any problems. I explained I was still experiencing severe pain in my chest and right arm. She noted it on my chart and left the room.

Dr. Walker entered the room and asked how I was doing. I explained the chronic pain in my chest and arm had worsened. He was mystified because he could not determine what was causing my pain, because my nerves had been severed during the surgical procedure he performed. Technically, my chest and arms should still have been numb. Once again I reminded him of my theory that the nerves had mended. He still insisted it was impossible, and I reminded him God has the last word, and I knew without a doubt he had mended my nerves.

Dr. Walker decided that rather than dismissing my theory, he would order a chest x-ray to see if there was any activity occurring in my chest. Therefore, I requested he also order a bone scan for my reassurance, which gave me comfort. I mentioned that I had been taking the narcotic pain medication Dr. Thomas had prescribed several years ago and that I had taken several pills, which relieved the pain. He agreed to write the prescription but also explained that the medication was addictive and that I should use it with caution. Meanwhile, the nurse gave me the information for the chest x-ray and bone scan scheduled at Westside Memorial Hospital.

On the morning of the tests, I was restless and having an anxiety attack. I decided to leave home earlier than planned. Michael would meet me later. When I finished registering, I was sent directly to radiology for a chest x-ray. I was informed that before I could have the x-ray and bone scan, I needed to have blood drawn to ensure I wasn't pregnant. My last cycle had been more than ten days. It was a state requirement for all women of childbearing ages to have the pregnancy test for the protection of the unborn baby.

I wasn't prepared to have my blood drawn and explained my phobia of needles. The nurse tried to comfort me by reassuring me she would only stick me once for both procedures. On the first attempt, the nurse did not draw any blood, because chemotherapy had left many of my veins unproductive. She tried again, and I began to cry hysterically and hyperventilate. She said that she understood the stress and anxiety I was experiencing and that she would make it as painless as possible. After everything was over, I had become so stressed out I had to lie down and wait forty-five minutes for the results.

After the pregnancy test results came back negative, it was time for the nuclear injection. The chest x-ray was scheduled first, and then the bone scan. The medicine would take two hours to circulate throughout my entire body. This was necessary to ensure every bone in my body was identified in case there was a problem. After the injection, Michael and I left the hospital and planned to return after lunch.

I arrived first at the hospital, and then Michael arrived a short time latter. The nurse began the bone scan promptly. It took two-and- a-half hours to completely scan my body. Michael sat patiently the entire time, watching my image as it appeared on the monitor. He was checking the monitor for "hot spots" that would indicate cancer. I asked him several times whether there were any hot spots; each time, he said no.

When the bone scan was completed, Michael returned to work.

I waited patiently in the lobby to make sure the radiologist was satisfied with the x-rays. The reading of the x-rays took an additional half an hour. While in the lobby, I noticed a comment box and took the opportunity to write a wonderful comment regarding the nurse. She was a godsend, and I was thankful for her presence.

The nurse finally entered the lobby and told me about her mother.

Her mother had succumbed to cancer. And she had taken care of her mother during her battle with cancer until she passed. Both of our eyes filled with tears as we embraced. I thanked her for being compassionate and understanding. She then told me the doctor was satisfied with the bone scan.

As I drove home, I prayed for a miracle. My follow-up appointment with Dr. Walker was scheduled for March 12, 2004. At that time he would discuss the test results. I knew without a doubt that before my follow-up, I would have imagined every negative scenario that could possibly occur. I nearly went out of my mind with worry. I continued to pray the test results were negative for cancer, although I needed to learn what was causing the pain. I hoped the pain could be managed with medication. I prayed to God to give me the strength and courage to handle the results of the bone scan, whatever they might be.

The day arrived for my appointment with Dr. Walker.

Michael accompanied me just in case there was earth-shattering news. I signed in and waited to be called. We were the only people in the waiting area. The nurse called my name and led us to an examining room and told us Dr. Walker would be with us shortly.

Several minutes passed before Dr. Walker entered the room. I could tell by his greeting everything was fine. He read the report and stated there were no signs of a recurrence of bone cancer. That was the most encouraging news I had received in a number of years.

The weight of the world had been lifted from my shoulders. We discussed how to manage the pain and decided that since the narcotic pain medication was working, I should continue to take it as needed.

Michael and I left the clinic, and we thanked God for the fantastic news. Neither Dr. Walker nor I could determine why the pain persisted, but now that I knew the pain was not related to bone cancer, I could live with it. I was euphoric at the joys of being cancer free! When I returned home, I immediately called my family and shared the wonderful news. I could finally relax and put my mind at ease.

Shortly after sharing my wonderful news with my mother, my day of celebration was disrupted when I learned Grace from Delfarms Corporation had succumbed to a recurrence of breast cancer. She was in her early sixties. I was sure her loved ones would miss her tremendously. I will always remember her kind words of wisdom and encouragement. Although we only knew each other for a season, she was an inspiration and will forever have a special place in my heart. Just thinking about Grace made me wonder if her coworker Lisa and her husband had resolved their situation; I pray God worked things out for them.

During the month of May, there were several cancer-awareness activities scheduled. For the first time, I participated in the Drive for Life fundraiser. The Drive for Life is sponsored by BMW. For every mile a BMW is driven, a dollar is donated to breast cancer research. The weather was beautiful, and everyone was anticipating an excellent turnout.

There were four series of BMWs to choose from, and I test drove all four vehicles. The dealership decorated a beautiful buffet for the participants. One has to love America; we get to test drive BMWs and have lunch at the same time. The BMW sponsors also allowed us to sign our names on a silver 700 Series that would travel around America during the fundraiser. I signed my name on the driver's side of the hood.

My next fundraiser was the American Cancer Society Relay for Life. The event started at 5:00 p.m. Saturday evening and ended at 5:00 a.m. Sunday morning. There were various sponsors participating. This was an enlightening experience, and I had the opportunity to meet many extraordinary and wonderful people who have survived cancer. When I listen to someone else's journey through life, I realize how blessed I am. Some cancer survivors are amazing, and we are true winners. All the cancer survivors introduced themselves and shared their brave stories.

There were people from all walks of life and of various ages. Cancer does not discriminate and has no boundaries.

Once we had walked the first lap, we were taken to an area that was reserved for the cancer survivors. A beautiful banquet had been prepared. Several groups from the performing arts community entertained us, including one group that put on a fashion show.

Everything was outstanding! Some of the dancers were as young as three years old. I was amazed at how many sponsors and volunteers supported the occasion. The event was inspiring.

After experiencing the fundraiser, I decided to become a volunteer with the American Cancer Society. I felt that with my knowledge and experience I could be of valuable assistance to someone. For many years I had debated becoming a volunteer. My mind was made up once I had attended the Reach to Recovery class; I knew it was the proper thing to do.

Becoming a volunteer has filled a void in my life and given my life meaning.

I believe my life has come full circle. I can recall that when I was assigned my first survivor, the satisfaction was fulfilling and confirmed in my heart I was doing God's will. I have learned many women are diagnosed with breast cancer and are alone without anyone with whom to discuss their concerns regarding this silent killer.

The telephone conversations are meaningful, and you can learn a significant amount of history from a survivor during a conversation. Once the conversation begins, I can hear the relief in their voices. Survivors need to know they are not the only ones that have been afflicted by this dreadful disease.

In the beginning, some women cannot even say the words *breast cancer*. Until they are comfortable with their diagnosis, I must refrain from using the term. Once they have realized it's fine to say "breast cancer," then they can begin the healing process. I believe that in order to heal, one must acknowledge the condition. Only then can you defeat the silent beast within.

The women who have lumpectomies are the blessed ones, but they still may require chemotherapy or radiation treatments along with regularly scheduled checkups to maintain their health. It is also imperative that they have yearly mammograms and pap smears.

I'm always honest with the survivors regarding my experiences with chemotherapy. I do not want anyone to think treatments are going to be like a walk in the park. I explain that some women tolerate the treatments exceptionally well, while others have a difficult time like the one I experienced. I also inform the survivors that if they are having any complications, they should notify their doctors immediately.

There is a variety of medications available these days to prevent anxiety, depression, fatigue, and nausea. I strongly recommend they take candy with them for their chemotherapy sessions. Candy helps to eliminate the horrible taste from the chemicals associated with chemo. I also suggest keeping soup and crackers on hand; it helped me when I became ill. My other recommendation to survivors is to have someone accompany them on their first session to see how well they tolerate the treatments.

Several days after a survivor has chemotherapy, I always follow up to see how well they tolerated the therapy. My heart is filled with joy when I hear them say they did not experience any side effects from chemotherapy or radiation treatments. I assure them they are fortunate.

Some survivors just need to express their emotional state regarding breast cancer or their reactions to the treatments. On several occasions I have met with a survivor for lunch to put a face with the voice and name. Once they see how normal I am, they finally realize their lives return to normal after treatment. It's important for them to remember treatments are temporary but are required to increase their chances of surviving breast cancer.

Chapter Eleven:

Second Recurrence

SEPTEMBER 9, 2005, WAS MY four-year oncology checkup with Dr. Walker. He entered the room and was his usual charming self. He asked his routine questions and began to examine me. Upon his examination, we discovered the lymph nodes on both sides of my neck were swollen and painful to the touch. I knew from the expression that filled his face something was terribly wrong. He said he needed to perform two needle biopsies. I began to cry hysterically as the nurse held my hand. Once Dr. Walker had finished, he told me the lab results would be ready in thirty minutes.

After the biopsies were performed, I immediately left Dr. Walker's office and went to the parking garage. I called Michael and explained the possibility of a second recurrence of breast cancer. He said he would be there soon. Next I called my dad and relayed the disappointing news.

I could hear the frustration in his voice. When I finished speaking with him, I called my sister Elaine, and she called Kimberly, and the three of us cried profusely as they tried to console me. Kimberly requested I not call our mother until she could be with her. When Michael arrived, I was still outside in the parking garage. He comforted me and told me not to worry.

Michael and I entered the office and waited for Dr. Walker's return. When he entered the room and took a seat, I knew without a doubt I was experiencing a recurrence. The only time Dr. Walker ever sits down is to deliver disheartening news. He was apologetic, but he informed me that I was indeed experiencing a second recurrence of breast cancer and that the cancer was in stage III. I immediately stood up from my seat, looked out the window, and began to stomp my right foot as tears rolled down my face.

I felt Michael's presence behind me, reassuring me God would see us through this recurrence. I asked Dr. Walker what my alternatives were for treating the cancer. He stated I needed to be under the care of an oncologist, because there were certain tests required that he could not order, as his specialty was oncology surgery.

He recommended Dr. Scott and explained she had become one the best oncologists in the city over the past five years. He notified her and asked if she could possibly see me the same day. Her office was located across the hall, so Michael and I met with her for consultation. She recommended I have a PET/CT scan, a bone scan, and a brain scan to determine if the cancer had metastasized to other locations in my body. The tests were scheduled for Monday. Once Michael and I had left Dr. Scott's office, I felt compelled to speak with Dr. Walker again. I needed to inform him that I was all right regarding the recurrence.

Later that evening, Kimberly called and informed me she was with our mother. When I explained my current situation to my mother, I began to cry hysterically. My mother's voice sounded as if her heart had been broken. She told me not to worry and that she and my sisters Elaine and Kimberly would arrive late Saturday night.

When morning arrived, I felt relived. I had prayed all night for God to give me the strength and perseverance I needed to get through this difficult time in my life. I thanked God for Michael. He is definitely my hero, and he has been with me through many storms. And he has never once complained. He is truly a godsend.

My family arrived late Saturday night and was ready for bed; they were exhausted from the fifteen-hour drive. On Sunday morning, my mother and sisters slept in while Michael and I attended church. During the morning worship, I was amazed; God had lifted my burdens. Through the entire service, all I could think about was Jesus and what He had done for me. Although this was a time of uncertainties in my life, I felt remarkably close to God. Having His love provided peace and tranquility.

After the service, we returned home, and I prepared breakfast as Michael entertained my mother and sisters. After breakfast I wanted to spend time alone with Jesus, and it felt as if I were floating on clouds above the mountains, and I had no fears. I played my gospel music and was in my own world. No one imposed upon me; I was experiencing true serenity.

Later that afternoon, as I was preparing dinner, our friends Johnnie, Gwen, Bernita, and Deirdre arrived for support. We embraced, and then I introduced them to my family. I entertained our guest briefly but returned to my room.

Periodically I would leave my room and engage in conversation, only to excuse myself after spending only a few minutes with our guests. Just the presence of my loved ones gave me the strength to continue my battle with breast cancer. Regardless of how this situation unfolds, I will never stop loving God, because He loved me first.

On Monday morning, as I prepared breakfast, Michael dressed for work. Later, Kimberly would accompany me to the clinic for the bone scan. My mother and Elaine would take the opportunity to relax. Kimberly and I arrived at the clinic. After signing the consent forms, I was given the nuclear injection. Once the medicine had circulated throughout my entire body, I was prepared for the bone scan. I instructed Kimberly on how to locate the hot spots on the scan. She sat patiently as I repeated the same questions regarding the hot spots. Once the scan had been completed, we waited for the radiologist to review the x-rays. The nurse finally notified us the doctor was satisfied with the x-rays and we could leave.

On Tuesday morning, as my family prepared to return home, I cooked breakfast; Michael dressed and prepared to go to the clinic with me for my MRI brain scan. After breakfast, everyone said his and her goodbyes. Michael and I sat in the driveway as Kimberly drove down the street.

We arrived at the clinic and waited a few minutes before I was called. The technician began the brain scan. The MRI equipment was quite noisy. Once the brain scan was complete, the technician began to process the film. We were able to view the x-rays. She said that according to her experience, my brain appeared to be perfectly healthy. I was elated upon hearing those words. I gathered my things and we left.

The next test scheduled was the PET/CT scan. These particular x-rays scan the organs and soft tissues. Because I am claustrophobic, Dr. Scott had given me a prescription for anxiety medication because the PET/CT scans were performed in a small enclosure.

On the morning of the PET/CT scan, I forgot to take the anxiety medication, but Michael felt I would do fine. When we arrived at the hospital, I informed the technician I was claustrophobic and had forgotten to take the anxiety medication. I asked her if it was possible for me to purchase two anxiety pills from the pharmacy; she felt I should do well without the medication.

Once injected with the nuclear medicine, I had to sit in a dark and cold room for an hour. When the hour had passed, I was taken to the MRI room, and the technician began explaining the procedure. Fifteen minutes into the test, I lost my composure and began hyperventilating and begging the technician to stop the procedure. I pleaded with her; I could not handle being confined. Ten more minutes passed, and Michael began to speak to me. He tried to calm me down, but it was useless: I just wanted out of the MRI machine.

The technician expressed concerns regarding the clarity of the film because of my constant moving; this might mean I would need to retake the tests. I lay there trembling from the coldness. I finally composed myself and spoke to the technician about whether I needed to retake the MRI. She could not answer that question without the radiologist reviewing the x-ray first. On the way home, I said nothing. I was in complete silence, hoping there would not be a need to have another MRI.

Three weeks later, it was time to see Dr. Scott to review the x-rays. I was traumatized and filled with disbelief.

The MRI revealed the cancer had metastasized to four areas in my body: lymph nodes, chest, both lungs, and my bloodstream. I was baffled as to how the cancer had ended up in my lungs. In my right lung, there was one tumor and the lung had begun to fill with fluid. In the left lung, there were numerous tumors. I could not comprehend why the cancer had not been detected until it had caused catastrophic damage.

My entire body became numb as I listened to Dr. Scott explain the methods for ridding my body of the breast cancer. She explained chemotherapy would be a last alternative. Then she mentioned there were numerous cancer treatments available that could be taken both orally and via injection.

She recommended we try a hormonal injection. The injection was designed to stop the body from producing estrogen; that would put me into menopause, stop the growth of the tumors, and perhaps even shrink the tumors. We would try this regiment for three months and repeat the MRI to determine if the tumors were responding to the therapy. Blood would be drawn every three weeks while checking the tumor markers to detect the levels of cancer remaining in my bloodstream.

In October 2005, Breast Cancer Awareness Month, I was invited to participate in two radio interviews for the local American Cancer Society. I also had the opportunity to take part in a local NBC special regarding surviving breast cancer. Medical research has proven that although Caucasian women are more susceptible to breast cancer than African American women because of genetics, they often survive the disease through early detection. However, African American women, who are less susceptible to the disease, die more often because their cancers are detected too late.

I am constantly speaking to young African American women about surviving breast cancer. I emphasize that acknowledging the disease is the first step in healing. I am certain if I had acknowledged there was a potential problem over a year ago, my situation would not be grave. I had all the signs of a recurrence and ignored them.

I developed a cough and never mentioned it to my doctors. As a result, the cough contributed to my right lung filling with fluid. I am not sure if I was in denial or just ignorant of the situation. Each time I spoke with my sister Kimberly, she would ask if I had spoken to my doctors regarding the cough. Each time, I told her I hadn't.

Although I had been battling breast cancer for eight years, my faith remained strong and I believed I would be healed of this recurrence. I fully understand healing sometimes takes time. I believe God tests our faith to determine our loyalty to Him. And each time we doubt Him, we take a step backward in the prayer lines.

Most people would be amazed at the number of people that believe having a disease and accepting the condition is a sign of sin and a lack of faith and therefore will not admit their bodies are ill. I refused to believe that notion, because innocent babies are born every day with cancer and other deadly diseases.

If God is still punishing us for our sins from the Old Testament, why did he sacrifice his only son so man could have eternal life with the Father! Nothing in this lifetime could make me believe I am being punished for sins that were committed centuries ago or perhaps before my birth through my parents. And if this is true, why did God decide to punish only me out of seven siblings?

I feel strongly that we all have dormant cancer cells in our bodies and that, for various reasons, the cancer cells become active. I believe this to be true because of the number of people diagnosed with the disease each year. In my opinion, if you do not want to be treated for the breast cancer or any other disease, make sure it is your decision and not someone else's influence. Cancer is unlike any other disease, and the damage it causes is almost irreversible as well as mentally devastating.

January 2006 was an unforgettable month. Michael's job required him to relocate to Louisiana for eleven months. I reassured him I would be fine and would travel there every other weekend. For the first time, I would deal with the recurrence without Michael accompanying me to my appointments. I hoped my next appointment with Dr. Scott would be a positive one.

During my appointment, Dr. Scott informed me the tumors had not responded to the therapy. She assessed the situation and recommended a different approach—an oral cancer medication, which is chemotherapy in pill. We hoped the medication would dry up the fluid in my right lung and shrink the tumors in both lungs. Radiation treatments would start in February to aid in shrinking the mass in my chest.

I left Dr. Scott's office and went across the hall for my appointment with Dr. Walker. While there I received some dreadful news. Dr. Walker informed me I was dying and predicted when my life was expected to expire. I was distraught by the distressing news. I recall wondering several years ago, when my cousin's wife Joyce passed, if I could handle knowing my life was coming to its finalization.

I literally went numb, and I realized my destiny was in God's hands.

Death is the final stage man goes through on his journey in this life, and it cannot be avoided. Therefore, we must all face the reality that someday the sun will set forever.

At first I could not comprehend why Dr. Walker felt obligated to share this shattering news, but as I drove home, I realized it was his professional obligation. This way I had the knowledge, in case I wanted to do anything significant, and this gave me the opportunity to get my affairs in order.

I regretted Michael was out of town, but I had to inform him of the catastrophic news. When I shared my disappointing news, he wanted to come home, but I told him not to. I planned to drive up on Monday. Just having his support was enough to reassure me everything would be all right. I decided to share my diagnosis only with my immediate family. It was bewildering trying to determine how to inform family and friends of the news of my expected death.

On Saturday night I went to bed early. I was in distress from the debilitating pain in my chest. By now the pain was constant, and the pain medication had failed. Sunday morning validated my faith in God. While lying in bed, experiencing excruciating pain in my chest, I prayed to God and asked Him to heal my body and remove the pain.

At that minute I began to slip into unconsciousness, but not before witnessing a spirit enter my body. I am not exactly sure how long the encounter lasted, but I do know for certain that when I awakened the pain had been removed and I was experiencing tranquility and my body was without pain.

God had confirmed I was still in His favor.

In February I had my first radiation treatment. After the initial consultation, the actual procedure took only five minutes. I felt positive the radiation treatments would shrink the mass in my chest. The only side effect encountered would be a radiation burn, which would heal once the treatments are completed.

Although I was without pain, my lung continued to fill with fluid, which indicated the chemotherapy medication had failed. In order for the medication to achieve its goal, the lung needed to remain dry. Dr. Scott and I decided it would be in my best interest to try another chemotherapy pill. I would also have a CT scan performed every three months to see if the tumors were responding to the new medication.

Four weeks into radiation treatments, the mass in my chest had shrunk.

Additionally, my right lung collapsed and filled with 1,800 ccs of fluid.

I was hospitalized for three days. We hoped the tumors would respond to the new medication once the lung was drained and had remained dry for a substantial amount of time. Ironically, I was still experiencing the chronic cough; and hoped the cough would cease in time. Meanwhile, I continued to pray for the miracle of being cancer-free. I continued to do my part by keeping all of my appointments and taking my medication properly every day.

During the first week in June, my lung continued to fill with fluid. My pulmonary doctor also revealed to me I was dying after analyzing the fluid from my lung. The fluid was cancerous. He later informed me of a procedure that could possibly eliminate the fluid and the cough. This would provide relief until I succumbed to the breast cancer. A cardiologist would insert a catheter into my lung. The procedure would allow me to drain the lung every day. This would ensure the lung remained dry and would enable the medication to work correctly.

The morning of the surgery, I had plenty of support to accompany Michael and me to the hospital. Bernita was there, along with one of the mothers from church. Mother Stephens had become my prayer warrior. Mother Stephens has supported me through some difficult times; Her presence alone was reassuring.

Before I was taken to the OR, the surgeon explained the possibility of the catheter remaining in my lung for the rest of my life. I became depressed at the thought of this tube becoming a permanent life support, but I figured I would do what it took to survive.

I remained in the hospital for two days before being discharged.

When I arrived home, I immediately removed the bandages to view the catheter. On seeing the catheter, I accepted the inevitable. I knew my health would start to deteriorate rapidly in a manner of time. As the days passed, I became depressed each time I drained my lung. I prayed to God and asked Him not to let me suffer. I had accepted my destiny, and I anticipated my death. This was the first time I believed Michael felt defenseless, and I am sure he expected my death as well.

Kimberly spoke with me each day to encourage me to live. Although she tried her best to conceal her fears of my dying, I could hear it in her tone each time she called. She knew I had given up because the thought of having the catheter in my lung was more than I could bear. She knew that because of my compulsive behavior the tube hanging out of my abdomen would drive me insane. I believe everything has a place, and the catheter did not belong in my lung.

The tube finalized the beginning of my demise.

My family wanted me to spend some quality time with them before my death. This would also allow Michael the opportunity to have some quality time for himself. Kimberly and my nephews Edward and Xyja drove down from Chicago to pick me up. I would stay for two weeks. We assumed this would be the last time my family would see me alive.

Even though I was ill during the entire visit, I enjoyed spending time with my loved ones on this final visit. Within two weeks of returning home, I was admitted back into the hospital because of more complications. I was exhausted, and my health was failing fast. I could not conceive of living the final stages of my life in and out of the hospital. I continue to pray to God not to let me suffer. I knew it would be just a matter of time before my sun would be setting forever.

Several weeks after being discharged from the hospital, when it was time to drain my lung, nothing came out of the catheter. I was terrified of the possibility that the fluid was unable to drain as a result of a blockage in the tube or in my lung. I immediately called the doctor and was told to come in for a chest x-ray.

After having the chest x-ray, I returned to the examining room.

When my doctor read the radiology report and viewed the x-rays, he was astounded. My lung was completely dry.

And because my lung remained dry, the catheter was removed in August, but the chronic cough persisted. I had lab work and a CT scan performed in September to determine the condition of my lungs.

The medication had begun to work and had shrunk the tumors in both lungs, but the cancer levels in my bloodstream had increased. Although the medication was working, I still continued to develop complications with my lung. By then I was vomiting every day, and at night I would wake up because I was suffocating. I had also lost over thirty pounds. My sprits were down, and I was ready to die.

Kimberly continued to call to motivate me. She always reminded me that I was my best advocate and that I needed to be persistent with my healthcare. She was determined I was going to survive.

Finally, after being hospitalized on several more occasions, the doctors discovered the cause of the chronic cough; it was an acute case of bronchitis. The bronchitis was discovered because of my persistence. My pulmonary doctor recommended a procedure using a bronchoscope. The procedure revealed my chest was consumed by mucus, which was vacuumed out. I was given antibiotics, both intravenously and orally. The series of treatments cleared up the infection and eventually the chronic cough.

Another year had passed. In October 2006, I was given another opportunity to participate in Breast Cancer Awareness Month.

My interview was with our local Fox 10 News. I felt privileged to share my story with thousands of viewers. Although a month has been set aside for breast cancer awareness, I am pleased that finding a cure for breast cancer is a priority in modern medical research.

I also continued to experience complications from the breast cancer and developed a cancerous nodule on the left side of my neck. The nodule started out the size of a pimple and grew to the size of a dime within six month. This incident led me to check my body regularly for suspicious pimples and bumps. I hope this will keep the cancer from metastasizing throughout my body.

After having the nodule removed from my neck, I elected to have a complete hysterectomy in November 2006. This procedure eliminated the production of estrogen in my body, lessening the chances of a third recurrence.

As usual, I was blessed to have my mother with me during this critical time. The hysterectomy was performed by an oncologist surgeon using the daVinci robot. The benefits of robotic surgery are that it is less invasive, it is more precise, and it requires less recovery time. Instead of having one large incision, I received five small incisions through which the uterus, ovaries, and fallopian tube were removed using glass tubes. I was overjoyed to learn there were no signs of ovarian or uterine cancer.

My last CT scan revealed the chemo medication was working.

The tumors had indeed begun to shrink in both lungs; my tumor markers were low for the first time in five years. But we discovered I had developed high blood pressure as a result of my failing lung.

On January 20, 2007, I was admitted back into the hospital by my pulmonary doctor. My blood pressure was dangerously high; I was also experiencing heart palpitations and exhaustion, and I could barely breathe or walk. I lost a substantial amount of weight, and I honestly expected to die in the hospital.

Around 5:00 p.m. my doctor entered my room with two large binders and took a seat. He did not speak for several minutes; he just looked and stared at Michael and me. To break the silence, I asked if the binders were my medical records, and he replied by saying yes. He then informed us that I was experiencing congestive heart failure.

He also mentioned my heart was only functioning at a 30% capacity.

He then asked if I was aware that two years ago my heart had been functioning at only 70% capacity.

I was dismayed that this vital information documented in my medical records had never been revealed to me. Michael and I were flabbergasted. Within the past five and a half years I had had at least fifteen PET/CT bone scans and brains scans and MRIs, and none of my doctors had ever thought to share this germane information with me. And what's ironic is that I had stopped requesting copies of my medical records.

The congestive heart failure was due to the long-term usage of chemotherapy, hormonal injections, and oral cancer medications. I fully understand that the long-term use of any medication causes side effects. I strongly believe I should have been informed when the PET/CT scans revealed the damage to my heart. The entire lower portion of my heart arteries are blocked, and even on medication, my heart will never again function at 100%.

Before being discharged, I determined I was going to fight to live my life to the fullest. For five and a half years I contemplated dying from breast cancer, only to learn I could have succumbed to complications from breast cancer: congestive heart failure, a collapsed lung, chronic bronchitis, and dramatic weight loss.

When I arrived home, the first thing I did was go outside and sit on my patio. This was the first time in years I had been able to go outside and breathe without any difficulties. It was serene listening to nature and feeling the cold air as it surrounded me. I thought about how wonderful life is!

Three years ago I was in the final stages of breast cancer; and informed by several physicians I was dying. Now, I am doing remarkably well and have transcended *From Midnight to Daylight* and I *"take the time to smell the roses."* I know this is made possible because of my faith, trust, and love for God and Christ. Being relentless in managing my healthcare along with listening to my sister Kimnberly advice had a tremendous effect on my surviving breast cancer. Although, I will never be that energectic person again, I plan to live a wonderful and fulfilling life and will enjoy each day as if it was my last.

Only God knows the exact date and hour which I shall succumb to death. Until that time, I will continue speaking to women regarding early detection of breast cancer. Perhaps by doing this, I can spare someone from becoming a victim to breast cancer.

Ladies we are our best advocate's. It is imperative to know your family medical history and paying attention to your body when it speaks to you listen. And if you are experiencing failing health, do not hesitate to seek additional medical advice and treatments. I am living proof that being relentless in managing your healthcare can extend your life.

"Early detection is the key to surviving breast cancer."

Chapter Twelve:

Notes From The Author

I WOULD LIKE TO TAKE the opportunity to share my reasons for writing *From Midnight to Daylight*. I strongly believe I have a story that is worthy to be shared with all women. These thirteen years of my life have led me to respect breast cancer. Breast cancer is a silent killer; it destroys everything in its path. This disease steals the lives of hundreds of thousands of women each year around the world.

Breast cancer is the number-two killer among women, with heart disease being number one.

Breast cancer is a silent killer, and it is regrettable that most women do not realize they have breast cancer until it's too late. If you are diagnosed with breast cancer, get treatment immediately. Do not procrastinate and take the chances of the cancer metastasizing. If contemplating reconstructive surgery, make arrangements to have the procedure performed immediately following the mastectomy if possible. Discuss any concerns regarding the procedure with your doctor.

I believe in the power of prayer for miracles, but I also acknowledge God gave doctors the knowledge and insight to assist Him in our earthly healing. Unfortunately, I know of far too many women who lost their lives prematurely as a result of breast cancer. They were told their church congregation could pray the cancer out of their bodies. Some were even told herbs would aid in ridding their bodies of cancer. In my opinion, you cannot have one without the other.

Therefore, prayer and medical treatments are both required in the healing of any disease.

I am confident herbs are powerful and possess healing powers and can aid in the prevention of certain diseases. We need to understand the definition of the word *prevention*, which means *to stop or keep from doing or happening; hinder.* One cannot prevent something that already exists.

One must also remember there are two types of tumors—benign and malignant. Benign tumors are usually fluid-filled cysts that can disappear, whereas malignant tumors are cancerous and must be treated radically to eliminate the disease from the body. Then there are at least seven different kinds of breast cancers; they affect each woman differently and must be treated radically to increase one's chances of surviving.

We are sometimes told not to acknowledge the breast cancer or some other illness that has invaded our bodies. I have this to say: God cannot heal you if you are in denial. Matthew, Luke, Mark, and John all stated every person Jesus healed was healed because those people professed a healing was needed for themselves or their loved ones. Not admitting you have breast cancer will not make it disappear. Acknowledging the disease can increase the chances of surviving this silent killer.

Some doctors are recommending chemotherapy or radiation before surgery; this is done to shrink the cancer, thereby improving one's chances of surviving the breast cancer. Chemotherapy has advanced tremendously since my first experiences. There are cancer blockers that aid in preventing recurrences of breast cancer. If an immediate family member has breast cancer, you can request to be tested for the breast cancer gene BRCA 1 and BRCA2 (Breast Reactive Cancer Antigen). This will determine if you are at high risk. All these methods can increase your chances of surviving breast cancer.

If you feel your doctor is not communicating with you, remember that you have the right to seek another doctor for a second opinion. Do not let your loyalty cost you your life. We must remember that we pay our doctors' salaries for the medical care we receive, whether or not we have medical insurance or receive assistance from state- or government-funded programs. Every insured person has a right to expect quality healthcare.

The American Cancer Society Foundation offers outreach programs that can assist in recovery and make the transition more tolerable. Do not try handling having breast cancer alone, because it is bigger than all of us. Encourage the women in your life to have regular mammograms and pap smears. Remember: Early detection is the key to life. Spread the word.

Chapter Thirteen:

Medical Definitions

BELOW ARE SOME UNFAMILIAR TERMS taken from my medical reports, defined as I understand them. However, medical terms have specific technical meanings, and I recommend asking your doctor or use a medical dictionary to understand the medical terminology being used.

Adjuvant therapy: a treatment given to assist the effects of another; for example, hormonal therapy or chemotherapy "adjuvant to surgery".

Adenocarcinama: a cancer that occurs in glandular tissue.

Adenoma: benign growth in the glandular tissue; a gland-like benign tumor.

Adenopathy: signs of disease in glands.

Androgen: a male sex hormone (also found in women) used to treat recurrent breast cancer.

Anemia: a deficiency of red blood cells, which causes pallor and fatigue.

Areola: the dark skin that surrounds the nipple of the breast.

Asymptomatic: having no symptoms.

Axilla: armpit.

Axillary: in the armpit; for example, the axillary lymph nodes removed during a radical mastectomy.

Benign: not cancerous.

Biopsy: removal of a small amount of tissue to be examined for signs of disease.

Bilateral: on both sides of the body.

Bone scan: a nuclear imaging method that gives important information about the bones.

BRCA2: Breast Reactive Cancer Antigen; a test for it can be performed to determine whether a person is at high risk for breast cancer.

Breast cancer: cancer that starts in the breast.

Breast implant: a sac of saline or other solution inserted into the breast under the skin to increase or restore its size.

Breast reconstruction: surgery that rebuilds the breast after mastectomy.

Breast reduction: surgery to make a breast smaller for reasons of comfort or appearance.

Bronchitis: acute or chronic inflammation of the bronchial tubes.

Bronchoscope: a tubular illuminated instrument used for inspecting the bronchial tubes.

Carcinoma: a malignant tumor located in the lining of an organ.

Chemotherapy: treatment with drugs to destroy cancer cells.

Chronic: marked by long duration or frequent recurrence.

Congestive heart failure: the heart is unable to maintain adequate circulation of blood in tissues of the body.

Connective tissue disease: various diseases such as rheumatoid arthritis, systemic lupus, etc. which affect ligaments, tendons or cartilage.

CT (computerized tomography) scan: a diagnostic method that creates a computerized image of the body to locate medical problems.

Cyst: a fluid-filled abnormal mass that is usually benign.

Diagnosis: identifying a disease by its signs or symptoms.

Duct: a hollow passage through which a gland's secretion passes Ductal carcinoma: cancer in the milk ducts of the breast.

Edema: build-up of fluid (lymph) in the tissues causing swelling.

Endocrine glands: glands that release hormones into the bloodstream.

Estrogen: a female sex hormone produced primarily by the ovaries.

Etiology: the cause of a disease.

Fibro-glandular densities: fibrous tissue in and around the milk glands in a breast.

Fibroma: a fibrous tumor.

Fibrosis: thickening or scarring of connective tissue.

Granuloma: mass of granulation tissue, usually occurring in response to infection, inflammation or a foreign substance.

HEENT: head, eyes, ears, nose and throat examination]].

Hemostasis: the stopping of the flow of blood.

Hepatosplenomegaly: enlargement of the liver and spleen.

Herpes zoster: shingles.

Implant: an artificial form used to restore the shape of an organ after surgery infiltrating: invasive.

Lesion: an abnormal change in structure or function of an organ; injury or damage.

Lumpectomy: surgery to remove cancerous tissue from the breast.

Lupus (lupus erythematosus): an inflammatory disease of the skin, which may also involve internal organs.

Lymph nodes (lymph glands): small glands that purify the colorless fluid drained from tissues (lymph) and manufacture white blood cells to add to it.

Malignancy: a cancerous tumor.

Mammogram: x-rays of the breasts to detect breast cancer.

Medial: towards the midline of the body.

Mediastinum: the middle membrane between the lungs.

Metastasis: transfer of disease from one part of the body to another; a secondary tumor at a distance from the primary site of the cancer; the spread of cancer.

Metastasize: to spread elsewhere in the body..

Micro-calcifications: small calcium deposits in tissue.

Modified radical mastectomy: surgery to remove the entire breast (see also Radical mastectomy).

MRI (magnetic resonance imaging): a nuclear diagnostic method in which a very detailed image is built up to show any signs of internal injury or disease.

Neoplasia: the presence of abnormal growths.

Neoplasm: an abnormal growth (tumor).

Nodule: a small, rounded lump or swelling (which may or may not be a tumor).

Palpable: detectable by touch; for example, a mass that can be felt in the breast.

Parenchyma: the functional portion of a gland as opposed to the connective tissues that support it.

Pathology: the study of diseases.

PET (positron-emission tomography) scan: a nuclear diagnostic technique that creates computerized color images of how internal organs are functioning

Port: is a small medical appliance that is installed beneath the skin around the collar bone. A catheter connects to the port to a vein for the chemotherapy injections.

Postmenopausal: having undergone menopause.

Progesterone: a female sex hormone that is released by the ovaries during the menstrual cycle.

Prosthesis: an artificial body part replacing a missing leg, arm, breast, etc.

Radical mastectomy: surgery to remove the entire breast and surrounding lymph nodes.

Recurrence: cancer that has come back after treatment.

Rheumatoid arthritis: a painful chronic, progressive disease causing inflammation and stiffening of the joints.

Sternum: the breastbone.

Supraclavicular: above the collarbone.

SWOG: Southwestern Oncology Group, an organization of oncology specialists]].

TRAMP flap (transverse abdominis musculo-peritoneal flap): removal of a flap of abdominal muscle to be used in breast reconstruction surgery.

Ultrasound: a diagnostic imaging method that uses ultrasonic pulses to show areas of different densities in the body.

My Beating Heart

Each morning when I awake, the first thing I see is my beating heart. It lets me know that I'm alive. The last thing that I see at night is my beating heart. It lets me know that my life has been spared for another day.

www.ingramcontent.com/pod-product-compliance
Lightning Source LLC
Chambersburg PA
CBHW021603280526
45784CB00001BA/477